MEDICAL AND SURGICAL EMERGENCIES

THE ABCDE APPROACH

Published in the UK by:-

Anshan Ltd
6 Newlands Road
Tunbridge Wells
Kent. TN4 9AT

Tel: +44 (0) 1892 557767
Fax: +44 (0) 1892 530358

e-mail: info@anshan.co.uk
web site: www.anshan.co.uk

© 2018 Anshan Ltd

ISBN: 978 1 848291 423

All rights reserved. No part of this publication may be reproduced, stored in a retrieval system, or transmitted in any form or by any means, electronic, mechanical, photocopying, recording or otherwise, without the prior written permission of the publisher.

The use of registered names, trademarks, etc, in this publication does not imply, even in the absence of a specific statement that such names are exempt from the relevant laws and regulations and therefore for general use.

British Library Cataloguing in Publication Data
A catalogue record for this book is available from the British Library.

Copy Editor: Andrew White
Cover Design: Elena Khoroshitseva and Emma Randall
Typeset by: Kerrypress Ltd
Printed by Cambrian Printers

MEDICAL AND SURGICAL EMERGENCIES

THE ABCDE APPROACH

Ruslan Zinchenko

Legal Disclaimer

The information provided in this book sets out the authors' opinion on how to approach medical and surgical emergencies of the type so described. The approach the authors have set out is one which they find useful, but which is not by any means universal and should not be taken as a rule to follow or a reference guide. Moreover, knowledge and best practice in the field of medicine are constantly changing and new research and experience may necessitate changes to the way in which medical treatment should be delivered. If you are faced with an unwell patient you should use your own knowledge, experience and common sense together with following your local hospital or professional guidelines on deciding the best course of action. You should seek senior or specialist help when unsure about what to do. In no event may any reliance be placed on the information provided in this book.

This book is intended as an information resource only. The information in this book is provided without any representations or warranties, expressed or implied, and in particular we do not warrant or represent that the medical information in this book will be up to date at the time of publishing, nor that it is true, accurate, complete, current or non-misleading. It is not intended to create a patient-doctor relationship.

To the fullest extent of the law, neither the authors nor publisher assume any liability for any injury and/or damage to persons or property as a matter of product liability, negligence or otherwise, or from the use to which any person puts any of the information contained within this book.

By purchasing and/or reading this book and any related content, you confirm and agree that the author (i) is not acting as an adviser in any capacity (ii) shall not be held to give (or have given) any advice, assurance, guarantee or other assessment as to the performance or likely outcome of any course of action described in this book and (iii) shall not be held liable for any decision made pursuant to or as a result of the contents of this book and any related content.

By purchasing or reading this book you are deemed to have agreed to this disclaimer and agree to be bound by it.

CONTENTS

Disclaimer iv
Acknowledgements vi
Preface vii
Reviewers page ix
Authors page xi

Introduction to the ABCDE approach 1
Respiratory Emergencies 23
Cardiac Emergencies 47
Gastrointestinal and Surgical Emergencies 83
Neurological Emergencies 121
Endocrine Emergencies 153
Electrolyte Emergencies 175
Oncological Emergencies 189
Haematological Emergencies 211
Poisoning Emergencies 223
Orthopaedic Emergencies 251
Obstetric and Gynaecological Emergencies 267
Paediatric Emergencies 289
Psychiatric Emergencies 321
ENT Emergencies 341
Skin Related Emergencies 357

ACKNOWLEDGEMENTS

Many people were involved in the writing of this book and it wouldn't have been as good as it is without their input. Firstly, I would like to thank all the co-authors, for writing excellent chapters on emergencies from different specialties. I am grateful to all the reviewers who helped to ensure that certain complex areas are spot on in terms of factual content. Elena, the designer, did a wonderful job, designing the book and implementing my ideas onto the screen. Finally, a big thank you to my family who were extremely supportive throughout the entire process of writing it.

PREFACE

The dialogue

Tim (first year clinical student) and Rus (final year medical student)

Tim: Hi Rus, how did finals go?
Rus: They were fine. Stressful, but that's to be expected. I am glad they're over.
Tim: I am dreading the end of the year, just because of the OSCE exams. Do you have any tips on how I should prepare?
Rus: It's all about practice. Get a group of colleagues together and just practice and act out different scenarios.
Tim: Yes, I've heard that, and will probably start doing that soon. Anyway, how do you feel about starting as a doctor?
Rus: The idea of starting work is exciting, but the idea of managing a critically unwell patient makes me nervous. I don't feel prepared to deal with emergencies.

This is the feeling that most final year medical students experience as they become doctors. Certainly, this is what was going through my mind and those of my friends and colleagues. We were taught the basics on how to approach a critically unwell patient, but none of us really felt prepared.

As we were revising for our OSCEs (Objective Structured Clinical Examination) and practising different scenarios of the critically unwell patient, it became apparent that there weren't many useful resources available. As a result we started creating our own DR ABCDE (Danger, Response, Airway, Breathing, Circulation, Disability, Everything else) scenarios to practice with.

After finals, we collated the materials created during our preparation for the clinical exams into a comprehensive resource on common medical and surgical emergencies for both students and junior doctors. When deciding on the format of the book, we decided to go with what we have found useful: scenario-based learning and discussions.

The content of the book includes topics that we would have personally found useful in medical school. It was then extensively edited and improved once we started working as junior doctors and, as a result, a lot of the cases are based on real life scenarios that we were involved in. Having worked through these scenarios ourselves, we believe that they did help prepare us for dealing with the critically unwell patients.

Having the clear structure demonstrated in this book to fall back on and these scenarios at the back of your mind will help you keep your cool and make clear well-considered decisions.

We would like to emphasize the fact that as a junior doctor working in a developed country you will never be expected to manage a critically unwell patient on your own. There will always be senior doctors whom you will be able to ask for advice. Therefore your role is to perform a brief but comprehensive assessment and to commence the initial management, prior to seeking help. This is what this book aims to teach the reader. As you become more experienced, the point at which you will seek help will get pushed back further and further. However, never forget that even the best of us require help sometimes.

The book is interactive and scenario-based. It is intended to be used in pairs or a group. Even though reading through the scenarios will certainly be of benefit to you, practise them with your colleagues and friends. Split yourself into an actor, a student or a doctor and an observer and work through the scenarios. This way you will be able to consolidate the knowledge that you already have.

When faced with a critically unwell patient for the first several times, it is very common for your mind to go blank. We hope that by practising these scenarios you will be more prepared when it comes to the real thing and the element of "muscle memory" will kick in, aiding you in making the right decisions in a timely fashion.

When writing this book we decided to highlight the importance of a good handover. At the end of each scenario you will be asked to hand over the patient to a specialty doctor who will take over their care and/or give you advice. The importance of clear and effective communication in medical emergencies is frequently underestimated and is poorly taught at both undergraduate and postgraduate levels. A good, concise handover leads to better continuity of patient care. It provides only the necessary facts, draws attention to the important findings, and prompts timely and appropriate intervention. However, just like any skill, it requires practice. Therefore throughout this book we would like you to practise handing over the patient at the end of each scenario. The format we suggest is SBAR (Situation, Background, Assessment, Recommendation), which is frequently taught in the UK. We have personally found it useful when attempting to structure our handover in our minds.

Each scenario is followed by an "In Brief" section, which asks a set of questions about the topic and was included for two reasons. Firstly, to replicate exam conditions in which the examiner asks questions at the end of each practical station. Secondly, to make you think more broadly and academically about the case. Make sure to make the most of these sections, taking the time to answer the questions before reviewing and discussing the answers provided.

The information in this book came from a variety of resources including lectures, bedside teaching sessions, real emergencies, seminars, journals, online articles, guidelines and books available to the medical community. This book is more about an approach rather than the latest set of guidelines. It is about getting you into the right state of mind and giving you the right set of mental tools. We do not claim that any of the content is our original idea or opinion. It is all based on our interpretation of what we were taught.

We have tried hard to keep the format of the cases throughout the book as constant as possible. However, the fact that each chapter was written by a different author means that there is some variability. We hope the reader will find this of benefit, since it gives an opportunity to learn about various individual styles.

As one can imagine writing a book takes time. Being a doctor also takes time, quite a lot of it actually. Therefore, writing this book in their spare time meant that the authors have sacrificed a lot and demonstrated incredible discipline and motivation.

It has been a useful experience for all of us, since it was the first time we have formally attempted to transfer the knowledge we have accumulated during our time as students to the future generations of doctors. Up until now it has been the opposite and we were on the receiving end. We are all extremely grateful for all the great teachers we had in our medical school, University College London, and all the authors of the countless textbooks we have used during our time as medical students. We believe this is finally our opportunity to give something back.

Dealing with emergencies systematically will become second nature to you with practice. When that happens, we will have achieved what we set out to do in this book. We hope you will find it useful in preparing for your examinations and the beginning of your career as a junior doctor.

Ruslan Zinchenko

REVIEWERS

Mr. Waseem Ahmed (ENT Surgery Specialty Registrar)
Guy's Hospital, London

- ENT Emergencies

Dr Malin Farnsworth (Consultant Physician)
St George's Hospital, London

- Respiratory Emergencies
- Cardiac Emergencies
- Neurological Emergencies
- Endocrine Emergencies
- Electrolyte Emergencies
- Oncological Emergencies

Dr. Maya Al-Memar (Obstetrics and Gynaecology Trainee)
Queen Charlotte's and Chelsea Hospital, London

- Obstetric and Gynaecological Emergencies

Dr Salman Naeem (Emergency Medicine Trainee)
Medway Maritime Hospital, Chatham, Kent

- Introduction to the ABCDE approach
- Haematological Emergencies
- Poisoning Emergencies
- Paediatric Emergencies
- Psychiatric Emergencies

Mr Iskandar Rakhimov (Clinical Fellow in General Surgery)
St. George's Hospital, London

- Gastrointestinal and Surgical Emergencies

Dr Ersong Shang (Foundation Trainee)
University College London Medical School

- Introduction to the ABCDE approach
- Respiratory Emergencies
- Cardiac Emergencies
- Gastrointestinal and Surgical Emergencies
- Neurological Emergencies
- Endocrine Emergencies
- Orthopaedic Emergencies

Mr Matthew Welck (Consultant Orthopaedic Surgeon)
Royal National Orthopaedic Hospital, Stanmore, Middlesex

- Orthopaedic Emergencies

CONTRIBUTORS – Alumni of University College London Medical School

Dr. Ruslan Zinchenko MBBS, BSc - Main Author

Dr. Elizabeth Minas MBBS, BA – Respiratory Emergencies

Dr. Weiguang Loh MBBS, BSc –Cardiac Emergencies

Dr. Janice Yu Ji Lee MBBS, BSc - Gastrointestinal and Surgical Emergencies

Dr. Yap Zhi Min MBBS, BSc - Neurological Emergencies

Dr. Chua Lee Wei Brian MBBS, BSc - Oncological Emergencies

Dr. Sana Owais Subhan MBBS, BSc - Haematological Emergencies and Paediatric Emergencies

Dr. Ersong Shang MBBS, BA – Poisoning Emergencies and reviewer

Dr. Gerard Gan MBBS, BSc - Orthopaedic Emergencies

Dr. Ruoxing Du MBBS, BSc - Obstetric and Gynaecological Emergencies

Dr. Samuel En Ci Quek MBBS, BSc - Paediatric Emergencies

Dr. Estelle Yeak MBBS, BSc - Psychiatric Emergencies and Dermatological Emergencies

Dr. Sahar Hamrang-Yousefi MBBS, BSc - Ear, Nose and Throat Emergencies and Dermatological Emergencies

Introduction to the ABCDE approach

Ruslan Zinchenko

Basic principles of dealing with acutely unwell patients

All acutely unwell patients should be approached in a systematic way so that nothing important is missed. The ABCDE approach is frequently taught in UK medical schools. It allows for early identification and treatment of the most life-threatening problems. It also requires the healthcare professional to frequently re-assess the patient to evaluate the effectiveness of the interventions.

For junior doctors an important part of the ABCDE approach is recognising the limits of their competence and seeking help from other members of the team early on, once life-threatening abnormalities have been identified. Frequently, the initial intervention will be a temporary "holding measure" which will buy some time to organise and initiate the appropriate definitive treatment.

In this chapter we will discuss how to approach an acutely unwell patient using the ABCDE approach.

The sequence is the following:
- Danger
- Response
- Airway
- Breathing
- Circulation
- Disability
- Exposure/Everything else

A useful way to approach any physiological system is:
- Look
- Feel
- Listen
- Measure
- Treat
- Reassess

Danger

Even though the notion of danger is frequently omitted from the traditional approach to the acutely unwell hospitalised patient, it is an important part of the assessment. Just like in Basic Life Support (BLS), your personal safety should always be your priority. You should always be aware of your surroundings and avoid placing yourself in dangerous situations.

Examples of dangers that you may encounter in the hospital include:
- Sharp injuries
- Aggressive patients or their relatives

Never put yourself at risk and ensure it is safe for you to carry out the assessment.

Response

This should be done by introducing yourself and asking the patient what the problem is. This will not only put the patient at ease, but will also give you valuable information about the patient's state. A patient who can talk to you is breathing through a patent airway, has a pulse and is perfusing their brain. Additionally, they can tell you what is wrong with them ie. "I am very short of breath doctor" or "I have terrible chest pain doctor".

A patient's level of consciousness can be quickly assessed with the AVPU tool: Alert (A), responds to voice (V), responds to pain (P) and unresponsive (U).

Box 1. Observations

Basic physiological parameters are an important and useful part of the assessment. Usually, worried nurses will mention the worsening patient observations when asking for an urgent review. If they don't - then you ask them for it. This will allow you to prioritise the patients that need to be seen first. A normal set of observations may suggest an overly-worried nurse and a patient who does not need your immediate attention. Alternatively, a worrying set of observations may suggest the underlying problem and could be an indication that you will need senior help from the start ie. putting out an arrest/peri-arrest call. In the UK the National Early Warning Score (NEWS) system is used to give a set of observations a score. The higher the score the more abnormal the set of observations.

Observation trends are more useful than a single set, and you should use them in establishing the diagnosis and deciding on the best management. A good example is a hypotensive patient. A blood pressure of 94/61 in a normotensive or a hypertensive patient is worrying. However, if the observation trend has been stable for the past 48 hours, you probably shouldn't start administering fluid challenges.

Normal observation ranges (however do always look at the trend!):
- Heart rate (HR) – 60 – 100 per minute
- Blood pressure (BP) – 120 – 140 (systolic); 60 – 80 (diastolic); however, this is highly variable
- Respiratory rate (RR) – 12-20 per minute
- O_2 saturations (SaO_2) – 94 – 98 % (on room air) or 88 – 92 % in patients with CO_2 retention
- Temperature – 36.5 °C (± 0.5)
- Urinary output (UO) – 0.5 – 1 ml/kg/hour

Airway

The assessment always starts by making sure the airway is patent. An obstructed airway is an emergency and should be dealt with immediately as it will quickly lead to hypoxia, brain damage and a cardiac arrest. The common causes of airway obstruction are:
- Foreign bodies, blood, fluids and vomit
- Swelling (e.g. anaphylaxis)
- Trauma
- Low GCS (≤8)

Do remember that as a general rule a talking patient has a patent airway.

Look for:
- Swelling and oedema of anaphylaxis
- Foreign bodies, fluids and vomit in the mouth (particularly if the patient is unconscious)
- Paradoxical chest and abdominal movements (see-saw respiration)
- Central cyanosis (late sign)

Feel for:
- Air movement
- Foreign bodies in the mouth
- Displaced trachea (trauma, tension pneumothorax and neck crepitus)

Listen for:
- Wheeze (asthma, COPD, pulmonary oedema, anaphylaxis)
- Stridor (foreign body, laryngeal oedema, croup, epiglottitis)
- Stertor (stroke)
- Gasping (foreign body)
- Snoring (collapsing airway with low GCS)
- Gurgling (fluid, vomit or blood in the airway)

Treat:
A simple **head-tilt-chin-lift** manoeuvre may be all that is needed to relieve the obstruction. However, if a cervical spine injury is suspected (e.g. following a road traffic accident) **a jaw thrust** manoeuvre should be performed instead.

If you suspect there to be a foreign body in the mouth you can remove it using **Magill forceps.** It is important to only place the tip of the forceps where you can see it, so that no foreign bodies are displaced further down. If the patient is vomiting or there is fluid/blood in the mouth you should put them onto their side. A Yankauer suction tip can also be used, but only suction what you can see.

Airway adjuncts can be useful in maintaining an airway that has already been opened with simple manoeuvres.

The **oropharyngeal airway** adjunct is used in patients with a reduced consciousness level as it can stimulate a strong gag reflex. It should be inserted upside down to avoid pushing back the tongue, and then turned back into its final position. Initially ask somebody to show you how it's done and then practise the insertion on a plastic model. As oropharyngeal adjuncts come in different sizes, you should be able to determine the right size for your patient. The length of the adjunct should be the same as the distance from the patient's incisors to the angle of the mandible.

The **nasopharyngeal airway** adjunct may be used if the patient remains conscious, as it is less likely to stimulate the gag reflex. The adjunct should be lubricated with some gel and then inserted into the bigger nostril aiming posteriorly towards the occipital bone rather than superiorly towards the nasal bones. You should apply a rotatory movement during the insertion. Similarly, practice inserting this on a plastic model first. Absolute contraindications to a nasopharyngeal airway are nasal and basal skull fractures.

Whilst on the hospital wards do familiarise yourself with all the above mentioned equipment as you may well need to use it in an emergency.

However, if the patient's airway is at risk, you should put out an arrest call prior to trying to manage it on your own as they will require a definitive airway and anaesthetic input.

Breathing

After securing the airway, a brief respiratory assessment should be performed. Severe hypoxia can quickly lead to brain death and a cardiac arrest and should therefore be addressed promptly. The common problems that can lead to respiratory compromise include:
- Tension pneumothorax, flail chest and open chest wounds
- Large pleural effusion
- Acute heart failure
- Severe asthma or infective exacerbation of COPD
- Severe pneumonia
- Overdose with opiates which suppress the respiratory drive
- Acute respiratory distress syndrome (ARDS) or transfusion associated lung injury (TRALI)

If the patient is talking to you in full sentences their respiratory function is probably adequate.

Look for:
- Respiratory distress
- Accessory muscle use
- Asymmetrical chest expansion or paradoxical chest movement
- Central cyanosis
- Lip pursing, nasal flaring

Feel for:
- Displaced trachea (tension pneumothorax, massive effusion, collapse)
- Asymmetrical chest expansion (flail chest, effusion, pneumothorax)
- Percussion dullness (effusion, consolidation) or hyperresonance (pneumothorax)

Listen:
- Wheeze (asthma, exacerbation of COPD)
- Crackles (pneumonia, congestive heart failure)
- Reduced air entry (pneumothorax, effusion)

Measure:
- Respiratory rate
- Normal target oxygen saturations are 94 – 98 %. In patients at risk of CO_2 retention (e.g. COPD) target saturations should be 88 – 92 %.

It is important to remember that pulse oximetry readings can be inaccurate in patients who are peripherally shut down, anaemic or have atrial fibrillation. Therefore an arterial gas should be done in acutely hypoxic patients.

Treat:
Ventilation is suboptimal in the supine position. Therefore patients who are conscious and are able to maintain their airway should be sat upright.

A hypoxic patient should be treated with oxygen. There are various devices available for oxygen delivery:
- **Nasal cannulae** – can deliver oxygen at 1 – 4 L/min, achieving a FiO_2 of 0.24 – 0.40. It is used for low-to-moderate oxygen therapy.
- **Simple facial mask** – can deliver oxygen at 5 – 8 L/min, achieving a FiO_2 of 0.35 – 0.50. It is used for moderate oxygen therapy.
- **Venturi mask** – can deliver oxygen at 4 – 12 L/min, achieving a FiO_2 of 0.24 – 0.60. It is used for targeted oxygen therapy and is useful in patients at risk of CO_2 retention.
- **Non-rebreathe mask** – can deliver oxygen at 10 – 15 L/min, achieving a FiO_2 of 0.60 - 0.80. It is used in critically ill patients.
- **Bag-valve mask** – used in peri-arrest/arrest situations in patients with inadequate respiratory effort and should be connected to high flow oxygen.

FiO$_2$ or fraction of inspired oxygen is the measure of oxygen concentration. The FiO$_2$ of ambient air is 0.21, because it contains 21 % of oxygen.

The maximum flow rate of a hospital oxygen tank is 15 L/min. As a general rule an increase in the flow rate by 1 L/min increases the FiO$_2$ by 4 %.

A patient with a cardiac arrest should be ventilated with a bag-valve mask attached to high flow oxygen (15 L/min) until they are stabilised. They will also benefit from early intubation.

All critically ill patients who present with reduced O$_2$ saturations should initially be given high flow oxygen at 10 – 15 L/min via a non-rebreathe (reservoir) mask aiming for target O$_2$ saturations of 94 – 98 %. Once the patient has been stabilised, the oxygen flow rate can be reduced ensuring that the saturations are maintained at 94 – 98 %. If the critically ill patient is at risk of hypercapnic respiratory failure they should still initially receive high flow oxygen, as hypoxia will kill them quicker than hypercapnia. The oxygen concentration should then be reduced, guided by regular arterial blood gases, looking at the pH and PaCO$_2$.

Patients who require high flow oxygen via a reservoir mask to maintain their oxygen saturations should be assessed by a senior clinician as soon as possible.

Unwell patients who are hypoxic but are not critically ill will require mild-to-moderate levels of supplemental oxygen depending on their oxygen saturations. In mild hypoxia, nasal cannula at 2 – 4 L/min should be used. If higher flow rates of oxygen are needed a simple facemask delivering 5 – 10 L/min can be used. If the above measures fail, then the non-rebreathe reservoir bag mask should be applied with high flow oxygen at 10 – 15 L/min.

Patients who present with an asthma attack or an exacerbation of COPD should also receive nebulisers (salbutamol, ipratropium). Patients with COPD or other illnesses, which put them at risk of hypercapnic respiratory failure, should have their target oxygen saturations at 88 – 92 %. This should be followed up with an arterial blood gas sample 30 – 60 min following the commencement of oxygen therapy, which should guide you in titrating further oxygen therapy .

If the patient is in type 2 respiratory failure (low PaO_2 and high $PaCO_2$), they may require non-invasive ventilation (NIV). Prior to commencement the patient and the type of NIV should be discussed with your seniors. Non-invasive ventilation assists the patient with breathing via a tightly fitting mask. Commonly used NIV in COPD patients with type 2 respiratory failure is Bi-level Positive Airway Pressure (BiPAP). These patients should be admitted to a high dependency unit (HDU) where they can be carefully monitored. Various BiPAP ventilation modes are beyond the scope of this book.

Further investigations

Arterial Blood Gas (ABG)

An arterial or even a venous blood gas is a useful test in an emergency, as it can tell you how unwell the patient is and point you in the direction of the underlying pathology. It can be quickly analysed on the ward without the need for a lab. Various blood gas sample machines calculate many different parameters. Here we will discuss the main ones.

1. pH
A good place to start the interpretation of an ABG is with the pH. The normal pH range is 7.35 – 7.45.
- A pH of <7.35 indicates acidosis
- A pH of >7.45 indicates alkalosis

2. PaO_2
Partial arterial oxygen pressure is a good way to identify impaired gas exchange and can only be measured on an ABG. The normal PaO_2 value is 10.6 – 13.3 kPa whilst breathing room air (FiO_2 0.21). However, do note that PaO_2 should rise on supplemental oxygen. A low or normal PaO_2 in a patient on supplemental oxygen suggests impaired gas exchange. A rough estimate is that the PaO_2 should be 10 kPa less than the % FiO_2. For example if the patient is given FiO_2 of 30 %, the PaO_2 should then be approximately 20 kPa.

A low PaO_2 with a normal $PaCO_2$ is known as type 1 respiratory failure and can occur in:
- Impaired gas exchange: pneumonia, acute respiratory distress syndrome
- Ventilation-perfusion mismatch: pulmonary embolism
- Reduced absolute O_2 pressure: at high altitudes

3. $PaCO_2$
Partial arterial pressure of carbon dioxide reflects the patient's respiratory function and is a good indicator of alveolar ventilation. The normal $PaCO_2$ value is 4.7 – 6 kPa.

A low PaCO$_2$ (<4.7 kPa) can lead to respiratory alkalosis and frequently results from hyperventilation. Common causes include:
- Anxiety and pain leading to hyperventilation
- Central nervous system lesions (e.g. stroke)
- Pulmonary embolism
- Initial stages of an asthma attack

A high PaCO$_2$ (>6.0 kPa) leads to respiratory acidosis and occurs in hypoventilation. A low PaO$_2$ with a high PaCO$_2$ is known as type 2 respiratory failure. Common causes include:
- Severe asthma attack and Chronic Obstructive Pulmonary Disease (COPD)
- Opioid overdose
- Severe pulmonary oedema
- Neuromuscular disorders (e.g. myasthenia gravis, motor neuron disease)
- Thoracic abnormalities (e.g. flail chest in trauma, severe scoliosis)
- Obesity
- Severe pneumonia

4. Serum bicarbonate ion (HCO$_3^-$)
The levels of serum HCO$_3^-$ aid in determining whether the underlying pathology is metabolic. The HCO$_3^-$ ions attempt to compensate for the changes in the blood pH. The normal HCO$_3^-$ levels are 22 – 28 mmol/L. A low HCO$_3^-$ suggests metabolic acidosis, whereas a high HCO$_3^-$ indicates metabolic alkalosis or compensation for a respiratory acid-base disorder.

Common causes of metabolic alkalosis include:
- Vomiting and surgical leak (e.g. post gastrojejunostomy)
- Hypokalaemia
- Bicarbonate administration
- Milk-alkali syndrome

Causes of metabolic acidosis are best classified in terms of the "anion gap", which represents the concentration of all the unmeasured anions in the blood. Most blood gas machines calculate the serum Na$^+$, K$^+$, Cl$^-$ and from these the anion gap can be calculated:

$$(Na^+ + K^+) - (HCO_3^- + Cl^-)$$

The normal value is 12 – 20 mmol/L. Sometimes K$^+$ is not included in the calculation and the normal value is then 8 – 16 mmol/L. Causes of metabolic acidosis can be divided into those that give a normal anion gap and those that give a raised anion gap on the blood gas.

The common causes of a normal anion gap metabolic acidosis include:
- Gastro-intestinal bicarbonate loss (e.g. diarrhoea, pancreatic fistula)
- Addison's disease
- Drugs (e.g. acetazolamide)
- Renal tubular acidosis
- Iatrogenic (e.g. overtreatment with NaCl)

The causes of raised anion gap metabolic acidosis can be further divided into those caused by exogenous and endogenous acids.

Endogenous acids are those that are produced in the body and lower the blood pH:
- Lactic acidosis (e.g. shock and sepsis)
- Uric acid (e.g. renal failure)
- Ketones (e.g. diabetic ketoacidosis)

Many blood gas machines also calculate the blood lactate levels (normally less than 2 mmol/L). A raised blood lactate concentration suggests that there is tissue hypoperfusion.

Exogenous acid metabolic acidosis can occur following an overdose with the following substances:
- Salicylates (e.g. aspirin)
- Ethylene glycol
- Methanol

5. Base
This describes the amount of "base" that will be required to compensate for the changes in the blood pH. The normal values are between -2 and + 2 mEq/L. A base deficit of less than -2 indicates acidosis and a base excess of more than +2 suggests metabolic alkalosis. Importantly, a base deficit of less than -10 mEq/L is a worrying feature and warrants a review by the critical care team.

Interpreting an ABG sample

Before interpreting a blood gas sample ensure that you check the patient's details, the date and time, whether it is an arterial or venous sample and the amount of oxygen the patient is on (FiO_2).

1. Look at the pH and determine whether it is an acidosis, normal or an alkalosis.

2. Look at the PaO_2 and $PaCO_2$ to determine the presence of type 1 or type 2 respiratory failure, and whether there is a respiratory acidosis or an alkalosis.

3. Look at the HCO_3^- to determine whether there is a metabolic acidosis or alkalosis.
   • Calculate the anion gap to differentiate between a normal and a raised anion gap metabolic acidosis.

4. Look at both the $PaCO_2$ and HCO_3^- to determine whether this is a mixed (both respiratory and metabolic) abnormality.

5. Evaluate the other parameters (SaO_2, lactate, glucose, Cl^- etc.) available on the blood gas sample.

6. Based on the patient's history, clinical findings and the ABG, come up with the most likely diagnosis and initiate the appropriate management.

Chest radiography

A chest radiograph can also be useful at confirming the clinical findings and helping you arrive at the diagnosis. It is good practice to interpret a chest radiograph systematically so that nothing gets missed. Always try to compare the current image to any previous imaging available to determine whether the abnormality is new. Conveniently, a similar approach to the assessment of an acutely unwell patient can be used – DRABCDE:

D - Demographics

Check the patient's details and the date the radiograph was done. Also determine whether it is a Posterior-Anterior (PA) or Anterior-Posterior (AP) film.

An AP x-ray is frequently performed in acutely unwell patients who are supine. The x-ray source is located in front of the patient, and the x-ray plate behind. However, in this view the mediastinal structures including the heart can appear larger and this should therefore be taken into consideration during interpretation.

A PA radiograph is performed with the x-ray source posteriorly and the plate at the front. In most cases the patients are asked to stand and wrap their arms around the machine to move the scapula out of view. These radiographs are easier to interpret as thoracic structures are better visualised.

R - Rotation Inspiration Penetration (RIP)

A **rotated** chest radiograph is difficult to interpret. Ensure that the medial clavicular heads are equidistant from the spinous processes of the vertebral bodies.

Without good **inspiration** the entire lung fields cannot be assessed. When assessing for adequate inspiration you should be able to count at least 6 anterior or 10 posterior ribs.

An under/over-**penetrated** chest radiograph is also difficult to interpret. The vertebral bodies impression should be visible behind the heart, and lung fields should have some markings.

A – Airway

Ensure that the trachea is central and is not being displaced or compressed. Common things that can displace the trachea are a large pleural effusion or a tension pneumothorax.

B – Breathing

Under this heading you should carefully examine both lungs. You can start by looking at the lung edge for air indicative of a pneumothorax. The heart border and the diaphragm should be distinct from the adherent lung, and if not this suggests a collapse or a consolidation.

Next examine the lung fields. You should note if there are any colour differences between the two lungs. White shadowing is almost always indicative of pathology. Describe the type of shadowing you see. It can be alveolar and poorly demarcated suggesting consolidation of pneumonia. A pneumonic consolidation will also frequently have air bronchograms throughout. Air bronchograms are bronchi, filled with air but surrounded with fluid-filled alveoli.

Nodular shadowing, which is frequently well demarcated, is more suggestive of a distinctive lesion such as benign or malignant mass. A well-demarcated lesion with fluid level is suggestive of a lung abscess or bullae.

Reticular shadowing describes multiple fine lines throughout the lung field, indicative of pulmonary oedema. Prominent vascular markings also support the diagnosis of pulmonary oedema, as do Kerley B lines (thin lines at the lung edges). Reticular-nodular shadowing suggests interstitial lung disease and fibrotic changes.

C – Circulation

Under this heading you should examine the heart and the related structures: the mediastinum and the hila. The mediastinum is at its widest at the level of the aortic arch and should not exceed 8 cm. If it is enlarged this could indicate aortic dissection. However, do note that chest radiographs have a poor sensitivity and specificity for aortic dissection. If it is suspected a CT angiogram should be requested.

The left hilum is always higher than the right. If the hila appear enlarged, this could be due to hilar lymphadenopathy, which commonly occurs in malignancies and infections. Bilateral hilar lymphadenopathy will cause a wide mediastinum and occurs in lymphoma, sarcoidosis, tuberculosis and lung cancers.

The normal heart size on a PA film should be less than 50% of the widest part of the thorax (rib to rib). An enlarged heart suggests cardiomegaly or a pericardial effusion. A normal heart can appear large on an AP film.

Finally the heart borders and the cardiophrenic angles should be assessed (the angles formed between the heart silhouette and the diaphragm). Blunting of the left heart border indicates pathology in the lingula, whereas blunting of the right heart border suggests an abnormality in the right middle lobe.

D – Diaphragm

The borders of the diaphragm should be clear. An indistinct diaphragmatic border indicates pathology in the lower lobes of the lungs. The costophrenic angles should also be clear, and blunting of these suggests a pleural effusion.

A pneumoperitoneum, as a result of bowel perforation, is suggested by a thin black line of air under the diaphragm.

E – Everything else

At the end you should take note of other features visible on a chest radiograph:
- Bones – are there any fractures? (e.g. a rib fracture causing a pneumothorax)
- Soft tissues – is there surgical emphysema? (which can compromise the airway if it occurs around the neck)
- Foreign bodies – central lines, nasogastric tubes, chest drains, ECG leads

There are 4 common acute presentations in which a chest radiograph is a useful aid to establishing the diagnosis:

1. **Infective exacerbation of COPD:**
    - Flattened diaphragm
    - Hyperinflated lungs (more than 6 anterior ribs visible)
    - Bullae throughout the lung fields
    - An area of alveolar consolidation

2. **Pneumonia:**
    - Poorly-defined alveolar shadowing or consolidation with air bronchograms
    - Blurring of the cardiophrenic angles and diaphragmatic or heart borders

3. **Pulmonary oedema:**
    - Cardiomegaly on a PA chest x-ray (more than 50 % of the widest part of the thorax)
    - Bilateral widespread reticular shadowing
    - Blunting of the costophrenic angles suggesting a pleural effusion (this could be large and extend to the upper lung zone.)
    - Kerley B lines
    - Prominent upper lobe vessels

4. **Pneumothorax:**
    - The lung field is separated from the thoracic wall by a black line of air. The thickness of the black line will vary, depending on the size of the pneumothorax.
    - Displacement of the trachea and the mediastinum and compression of the whole lung in a tension pneumothorax. It is often said that this should be a clinical diagnosis that requires immediate treatment and shouldn't be picked up on a chest radiograph.

Circulation

A brief cardiovascular assessment should be carried out next. Common cardiovascular problems that are encountered in acutely unwell patients are:
- Hypotension and shock - hypovolaemic, septic, cardiogenic etc.
- Cardiac arrhythmias
- Fluid overload

Look for:
- Dyspnoea
- Oedema
- Dry mucous membranes
- Raised JVP
- Diaphoresis

Feel for:
- Cold peripheries
- Warm and clammy
- Pulse character and rhythm
- Skin turgor
- Pitting oedema

Listen for:
- Heart sounds
- Lung bases for crackles

Measure:
- Heart rate (HR)
- Blood pressure (BP)
- Temperature
- Urinary output (UO)
- Capillary refill time (CRT) (<2 s)

Treat:

Under this section the most common treatment you will be administering is intravenous fluids. Acutely unwell patients who present with shock, hypovolaemia or acute kidney injury will require intravenous fluid resuscitation. This seemingly simple treatment is frequently improperly taught in medical schools and as a result poorly understood by medical students and junior doctors alike. However, appropriate fluid therapy improves patient outcomes and you should therefore be comfortable with prescribing fluids in acutely unwell patients.

The daily fluid requirement of an average person is 30 ml/kg/24 hr. So with a body weight of 70 kg, the daily requirement would be 70 x 30 = 2,100 ml. However, one should also consider insensible fluid losses associated with vomiting, diarrhoea, fever etc.

The daily electrolyte requirement is approximately 2–4 mmol/kg of Na^+, K^+ and Cl^-. The daily glucose requirement varies between 50 – 100 g.

The common types of fluids used in hospital include:
- **Sodium Chloride 0.9 %** – this is probably the most frequently administered fluid. It contains 154 mmol/l of Na^+ and Cl^-.
- **Hartmann's solution** – second most commonly used fluid. It contains Na^+ – 131 mmol/l, K^+ – 5 mmol/l, Cl^- – 111 mmol/l, Ca^{2+} - 2mmol/l, Lactate - 29 mmol/l.
- **Glucose 5 %** – commonly used to treat hypernatraemia and contains 5 g of glucose per 100 ml.
- **Colloid** – known as a plasma expander, which contains macromolecules that increase oncotic pressure ensuring the fluid stays intravascularly. It is rarely used.

Frequently, potassium chloride will have to be added to the intravenous fluids. The maximum rate of K^+ that can be administered on a regular ward should not exceed 10 mmol/h because of the risk of inducing cardiac arrhythmias.

There is an ongoing debate about whether a crystalloid or a colloid is a better resuscitation fluid. The physiological mechanism of action of colloid makes it a better resuscitation fluid. However, studies have failed to show its significant advantage over normal saline. Furthermore, it can trigger anaphylactic reactions, it may be difficult to offload in case of fluid overload, it can prolong clotting times and in acutely dehydrated patients can contribute to kidney injury.

Acutely unwell patients who are fluid depleted, regardless of the underlying cause, may demonstrate the following:
- Tachycardia
- Postural blood pressure drop initially and hypotension later on
- Reduced urine output or anuria
- Increased capillary refill time
- Cold extremities

Acutely unwell patients who are hypotensive will initially require a fluid challenge. Usually with 250 - 500 mL of a crystalloid such as sodium chloride 0.9 % or Hartmann's solution given over 15 minutes or less. This should be done with caution in patients at risk of heart failure or those who are elderly and frail. If the patient responds to the fluid challenge: their heart rate goes down and the blood pressure with the urinary output go up, they should be written up for more fluids, adjusted according to the individual's needs and fluid status. These patients should be frequently monitored and reassessed and may require a catheter insertion for a more accurate fluid balance.

If the patient fails to respond to the initial fluid challenge, a further 500 ml should be given. This should be repeated up to 2000 ml. If the patient still fails to respond, you should seek senior help as soon as possible as they may require critical care review and ionotropic support.

If you suspect that a patient is bleeding they may well require a blood transfusion. It is important to clearly label the blood sample by the bedside before sending it off to the lab. There are two ways blood gets analysed in the lab. During a group and save (G&S) the blood gets analysed for ABO and RhD antigens and the common red cell antibodies. If the patient has previously received a blood transfusion and it was more than 72 hours ago, they will require a new G&S sample as they could have developed new red cell antibodies. The second type of analysis is a crossmatch. During a crossmatch the blood is analysed similarly to G&S but is also screened for antibodies against compatible stored blood products.

> In an emergency blood can be issued without a full crossmatch but this carries a higher risk of transfusion reactions. During a major haemorrhage O-negative blood can be given during the initial stages until a full crossmatch has been done.

Further investigations

Electrocardiogram (ECG)

An electro-cardiogram (ECG) will be frequently required under this section of the assessment. An ECG should be performed in all patients presenting with cardiovascular symptoms and ideally compared to any previous ECGs to identify any new changes.

It is important to evaluate an ECG systematically in order to avoid missing anything important. With time you will develop your own method, however here are several ways you can approach an ECG.

1. Patient details
Be sure that you are interpreting the ECG of the correct patient and that the date and the time are known. Have a look at any previous ECGs available. Ensure that the ECG was performed under correct settings. The speed of the paper trace should be 25 mm/s and in the standard voltage calibration 1mV should be equal to 10mm.

2. Rate and Rhythm
If the ECG machine is set to 25 mm/s each large square is 5 mm in length and represents a time interval of 0.2 seconds. Each small square is 1 mm in length and represents a time interval of 0.04 seconds.

The heart rate can be calculated by counting the number of large squares between each QRS complex, and then dividing 300 by this number. For example, if there are 3 large squares between each QRS complex, the heart rate will be 100 beats per minute (300/3 = 100). Alternatively, you can count the number of QRS complexes in 10s and multiply this by 6 (works better with an irregular rhythm).

Next, determine the rhythm. A P-wave should precede each QRS complex, which should occur at regular intervals. An easy way to see if the QRS complexes are regular is to take a white sheet of paper and mark the initial QRS complexes on the edge. Then move the marked piece of paper further along the ECG to determine whether the subsequent QRS complexes correspond to the initial ones.

3. Axis
The cardiac axis can be easily determined by looking at the limb leads I, II, and III. A positive QRS complex deflection in lead I (dominant R-wave) and a negative deflection (dominant S-waves) in leads II and III indicates left axis deviation. A positive QRS complex deflection in lead III and a negative deflection in leads I and II suggests right axis deviation. Any other combination of the QRS complexes indicates a normal cardiac axis.

4. P-wave
Next you should evaluate the P-wave. An absent P-wave suggests atrial fibrillation or atrial flutter. Abnormally shaped P-waves can occur in various atrial tachyarrhythmias or with structural defects of the atria such as hypertrophy.

5. PR interval
The normal length of the PR interval is 0.12 – 0.2 seconds, which corresponds to 3 – 5 small squares. The PR interval is prolonged in various forms of heart block and shortened in junctional tachycardias, ectopic atrial foci and Wolff–Parkinson–White (WPW) syndrome (due to an accessory conduction pathway, known as the bundle of Kent between the atria and the ventricles). In WPW syndrome the PR interval is shortened as a result of a delta wave, which represents a slurred upstroke before the QRS complex.

6. QRS complex
The normal QRS complex is less than 0.12 seconds or 3 small squares. A widened QRS complex occurs if the rhythm originates in the ventricles or if there is a bundle branch block.

7. ST segment
The ST segment should be at the same level as the ECG baseline. An elevation of more than 1 mm in the limb leads and 2 mm in the chest leads suggest myocardial infarction. ST depression of more than 0.5 mm suggests myocardial ischaemia. An upward J-wave (Osborn wave) occurs immediately after the QRS complex in hypothermia and hypercalcaemia.

8. QT interval
The QT interval is found between the start of the Q wave and the end of the T wave. The normal QT interval is less than 0.42 seconds in males and 0.44 seconds in females. A prolonged QT interval increases the risk of developing ventricular arrhythmias.

9. T-wave
T-wave inversion, particularly in leads I, II and V4 – V6 suggests myocardial ischaemia. However, it is important to remember that T wave inversion in leads III, aVR, and V1 in association with a predominantly negative QRS complex is normal.

Tall or peaked T waves are associated with hyperkalaemia. This can deteriorate into ventricular fibrillation and should therefore be treated as an emergency. On the contrary, hypokalaemia leads to flattened T-waves and can also cause U-waves to appear after T-waves.

Important ECG findings

You should never miss the following diagnoses on an ECG:

1. Ventricular tachycardia
    - Broad and regular QRS complexes
    - Rate of 110 – 200 beats per minute

2. Complete heart block
    - Severe bradycardia
    - Dissociation of P-waves and QRS complexes (no conduction via AV node)

3. ST elevation/depression
    - ST segment elevation of >1 mm in limb leads or >2 mm in chest leads (STEMI)
    - ST segment depression (NSTEMI)

4. New onset left bundle branch block (suggestive of acute myocardial infarction)
    - Wide QRS complex
    - QRS W pattern in V1
    - QRS M pattern and absence of a Q-wave in leads in V5 – 6

When presented with a bradyarrhythmia or a tachyarrhythmia on an ECG, the first step should be to ensure that the patient is haemodynamically stable. A patient who is drowsy or unresponsive, complains of chest pain or shortness of breath, or is hypotensive with a systolic BP of <90 is cardiovascularly compromised and requires immediate cardioversion or external pacing. You should get in touch with your seniors immediately or put out an arrest call.

5. Supraventricular tachycardia
    - Narrow QRS complex
    - Absence of P-waves
    - Fast rate >150

6. Ventricular fibrillation
    - Chaotic irregular deflections on the ECG strip
    - No visible P-waves, QRS complexes or T-waves

There are multiple bradyarrhythmias and tachyarrhythmias, which, if the patient is cardiovascularly stable, require specific treatments. These are beyond the scope of this chapter. Following a detailed assessment you should discuss the patient with your senior and initiate the appropriate management plan.

Disability

1) AVPU/Glasgow Coma Scale (GCS)

As previously mentioned, the patient's cognition can be assessed using the AVPU scale:
- Alert
- Voice (responds to)
- Pain (responds to)
- Unresponsive

The AVPU scale is useful as a triage tool. A previously well and alert patient who suddenly becomes only responsive to voice, pain or unresponsive should be assessed immediately.

You should then always perform a Glasgow Coma Scale (GCS) assessment:

Eyes
- 4 – eyes opening spontaneously
- 3 – eyes open to voice
- 2 – eyes open to pain
- 1 – eyes do not open

Voice
- 5 – talking and orientated to time and place
- 4 – talking but confused
- 3 – using inappropriate words
- 2 – mumbles sounds
- 1 – quiet

Movement
- 6 – obeys commands
- 5 – localises pain
- 4 – withdraws from pain
- 3 – abnormally flexes to pain
- 2 – extends to pain
- 1 – doesn't move

Following a head injury any deterioration in the patient's GCS should be taken seriously and the patient should be immediately assessed. In a patient previously scoring 15/15 a CT head should be done if the GCS becomes 13/15 or less. In patients with a persistent GCS of 14/15 a CT head should also be considered. In patients with previously abnormal GCS scores, a CT head should be done if the GCS score drops by 2 or more points. If a drop in one point persists, a CT head should also be considered. If unsure, do call the on call radiologist or your senior to discuss the case.

A GCS score of 8 or less suggests that the patient's airway is at risk and that a definitive airway may be required. All patients with a GCS of 8 or less should be assessed by an anaesthetist as soon as possible.

2) Blood glucose
All acutely unwell patients who are scoring less than 15 on the GCS should have their capillary blood glucose checked. A level of between 4 – 10 mmol/L should be considered normal in an emergency. Any hypo-/ or hyperglycaemia should then be appropriately managed.

3) Pupils
All acutely unwell patients who are scoring less than 15 on the GCS should have their pupil reaction to light checked. Any abnormality in the pupillary reaction should be taken seriously and must be immediately discussed with your seniors. The patient may require urgent CT head imaging. An abnormally reactive pupil in an acutely unwell patient may indicate:
- Brainstem pathology
- Raised intracranial pressure

If clinically appropriate a brief neurological examination should be performed. This should at least include proximal and distal power assessment and reflexes.

Exposure

Having now done the basic assessment to identify any life-threatening issues, under this section you should consider carrying out any further examinations and investigations, which would aid you in making a diagnosis or initiating the appropriate treatment.

These can include:
- Further blood tests (FBC, U&Es, TFTs, Troponin, BNP, blood cultures etc.)
- Imaging (abdominal x-ray, limb x-ray, angiography, CT scans)
- Oesophagogastroduodenoscopy (OGD)

The Effective Handover

A clear and concise handover leads to better continuity of patient care. It should provide only the necessary facts, draw attention to the important findings and prompt timely and appropriate intervention.

The SBAR communication tool, (developed by the health care consortium *Kaiser Permanente*, who adapted it from the US Navy), is commonly used to facilitate an effective and efficient clinical handover. It stands for:

Situation - patient details and a one sentence summary of the problem

Background – relevant background information on the patient

Assessment – relevant clinical findings, investigation results and initial interventions

Recommendation – statement of what further management is required

Respiratory Emergencies

Elizabeth Minas and Ruslan Zinchenko

Tension Pneumothorax	24
Pneumonia	28
Infective Exacerbation of COPD	32
Acute Exacerbation of Asthma	36
Pulmonary Embolism (PE)	40

Case 1 – **Tension Pneumothorax**

You are a Foundation Year 1 doctor working on the acute medical ward. You are asked to urgently attend to Mr Adam Green, who has suddenly become more breathless, dropped his oxygen saturations and is now less responsive. Mr Green was admitted yesterday with an infective exacerbation of COPD and since this morning he has been complaining of some right-sided chest pain.

Please conduct an A to E assessment of Mr Green and commence the initial management.

Latest observations:
HR: 123 BP: 93/51 RR: 29 SaO$_2$: 83% (2 L O$_2$); Temp: 37.0 °C; U/O: NA

Danger
It is safe to approach Mr Green.

Response
Mr Green is responsive to voice. Consider calling for senior help at this point.

Airway
Look – nothing in the mouth
Feel – trachea deviated to the left
Listen – rapid laboured breathing
Treat – the patient is maintaining his airway, move on

Breathing
Look – cyanosed, rapid laboured breathing, using accessory muscles
Feel (if not felt previously) – trachea deviated to the left; right hemithorax is hyperinflated with reduced expansion. Hyperresonant on percussion.
Listen – no air entry in the right hemithorax
Measure – RR 29, SaO_2 83 % (2 L O_2 via nasal cannula)
Treat – give high flow oxygen to maintain SaO_2 between 94–98 % since the patient is acutely unwell. It is important to recognise the right-sided tension pneumothorax and urgently treat it with needle decompression (See box 1).
Reassess – trachea is now central; his saturations rise to 94 % on 15 L and RR is 23

Further investigations (only following the decompression of the tension pneumothorax):
- ABG (titrate FiO_2 accordingly)
- Chest radiograph - demonstrates right-sided pneumothorax

Circulation

Look – pale, clammy, distressed, JVP raised
Feel – sweaty, cold peripheries, apex beat is displaced to the left, CRT = 3 seconds
Listen – heart sounds normal, parasternal heave
Measure – HR: 123, regular; BP: 93/51; temp: 37.0 °C
Treat – obtain IV access and decompress the tension pneumothorax.
Reassess – Following the decompression: HR 109, BP 110/74, temp 37.0 °C

Further investigations:
- ECG monitoring

Disability

AVPU – responds to voice/GCS 12 (E3, V4, M5)
Capillary blood glucose – 6.0 mmol/L
Pupils – equal and reactive to light

Exposure

Fully expose the patient and perform a detailed secondary examination

Hand over the patient to Dr Patel (Medical SpR on call)

Situation – My name is Dr _____ and I am the F1 on the acute medical ward. I have been called to assess Mr Green who has become suddenly short of breath and less responsive. I suspect he had a tension pneumothorax.

Background – Mr Green was admitted yesterday with an infective exacerbation of COPD, for which he is receiving intravenous antibiotics.

Assessment – On initial assessment the patient was responsive to voice and in respiratory distress. His observations were HR: 123, BP: 93/51, RR: 29, SaO_2: 83 % (on 2 L O_2), temp 37.0 °C. He was cyanosed, with rapid laboured breathing and his trachea was deviated to the left. The right side of his chest was hyperinflated with reduced expansion. It was hyper-resonant on percussion. There was no air entry in the right lung. I suspected a right-sided tension pneumothorax and inserted a needle into the right second intercostal space in the midclavicular line. This has led to an improvement in his clinical state. A chest x-ray demonstrated a right-sided pneumothorax.

Recommendation – I would like you to review this patient and consider performing a chest tube thoracostomy as a more permanent solution for his pneumothorax.

Box 1. Management of a tension pneumothorax

Insert a needle into the second intercostal space along the midclavicular line, just above the third rib. The needle should enter the intrapleural space and release the pressure. It is important to avoid the intercostal groove when placing the needle. An experienced clinician should then perform a chest-tube thoracostomy and the patient transferred to a high dependency area.

Tension pneumothorax in brief:

1. What is the pathophysiology of a tension pneumothorax?
- During a pneumothorax air can collect within the pleural space. This happens as a result of an abnormal connection between the alveoli and the pleural space. Since the alveolar pressure is normally higher than the intrapleural pressure, the air escapes following the pressure gradient.
- A tension pneumothorax occurs when the air gets trapped and accumulates within the pleural space leading to a rise in the intrapleural pressure. The build up of pressure goes on to exceed the alveolar pressure and leads to the compression of the lung and displacement of the great vessels. This leads to respiratory failure and cardiorespiratory arrest.

2. What are the risk factors for a pneumothorax?
The general risk factors include being male, having a tall and slender body build, smoking, lung disease, mechanical ventilation and past medical history of pneumothoraces.

Respiratory conditions that predispose to the development of a pneumothorax include:
- Chest wall trauma
- Asthma and COPD
- Tuberculosis
- Cystic fibrosis
- Pneumocystis jirovecii infection

What are the management options of a recurrent pneumothorax?
The usual recommended management is with a video-assisted thoracoscopy with stapling of the air leak as well as pleurodesis. Pleurodesis may be mechanical or chemical (using talc). These patients should have a chest drain placed whilst awaiting definitive management.

Case 2 – **Pneumonia**

You are a Foundation Year 2 doctor working in the emergency department. Ms Claire Jones, a 67 year old retired school teacher, presents with a temperature, a cough productive of yellow sputum and shortness of breath. Whilst you are looking up some blood results on the system, a nurse calls for your assistance, as Ms Jones has become very dyspnoeic and tachypnoeic.

Please conduct an A to E assessment of Ms Jones and commence the initial management.

Latest observations:
HR 110; BP 95/58; RR 31; SaO_2 89 % (room air); temp 38.7 °C U/O: NA

Danger

It is safe to approach the patient.

Response

Ms Jones appears delirious and responds to you with a nod and utters only a couple of words. She is having difficulty catching her breath.

Airway

Ms Jones is able to speak, so you are reassured that the airway is patent.

Breathing

Look – distressed, breathing rapidly and leaning forward, as she tries to catch her breath
Feel – the trachea is central and chest expansion is normal; there is dullness to percussion on the right lung base
Listen – you hear crackles on the right lung base on auscultation
Measure – RR 31, SaO_2 89 % on room air
Treat – give high flow oxygen via non-rebreathe mask to maintain SaO_2 between 94–98 % and adjust flow rate accordingly
Reassess – her saturations rise to 94 % and RR is now 25

Further investigations:
- Chest x-ray - demonstrates consolidation in the right lower lung zone
- Sputum microscopy and culture, urine antigens
- ABG - demonstrates type 1 respiratory failure with lactic acidosis

Circulation

Look – appears sweaty and cyanosed
Feel – regular fast pulse; she feels warm to touch
Listen – heart sounds normal
Measure – HR 110, BP 95/58, CRT <2 seconds; UO: not available; temp 38.7 °C.
Treat – obtain IV access; commence IV fluids (fluid challenge of 500 ml of Hartmann's or NaCl 0.9 %); commence paracetamol to address the pyrexia. Commence empirical antibiotics as per hospital guidelines.
Reassess – HR 90 bpm, BP rises to 110/70

Further investigations:
- Bloods (FBC, U&E, LFTs, CRP)
- Blood cultures
- Calculate the CURB 65 score for guidance on further management (her urea is 8 mmol/L)

Disability

AVPU – alert/GCS 13 (E4, V3, M6)
Capillary blood glucose – 5.5 mmol/L
Pupils – equal and reactive to light

Exposure

Fully expose the patient and perform a detailed secondary examinatio

Hand over to Dr Robinson (Medical SpR on call)

Situation – Good afternoon Dr Robinson I am _____ the F2 doctor working in the emergency department. I was asked to see Ms Claire Jones, a 67-year-old lady who I suspect has sepsis secondary to severe community acquired pneumonia.

Background – She presented with a cough that was causing her to feel severely short of breath.

Assessment – On examination, she appeared confused and very dyspnoeic. She had crackles and dullness to percussion in the right lung base. Her RR was 31 and she was saturating at 89 % on room air. Her heart rate was 110 bpm and her blood pressure was 95/58. Her temperature was 38.7 °C. I placed her on high flow oxygen through a non-rebreathe mask and her saturations improved to 94 %. I administered a 500 ml fluid challenge of Hartmann's solution and her BP increased to 110/70 and her HR came down to 90 bpm. I also gave her 1 gram of IV paracetamol for her pyrexia. I have ordered a chest x-ray, taken blood cultures and baseline bloods, performed an ABG, which showed type 1 respiratory failure, and commenced empirical antibiotics as per hospital guidelines.

Recommendation – I have been unable to obtain a full history, as she is dyspnoeic and has not yet been clerked. My impression is that she is suffering from a severe community-acquired pneumonia with a CURB 65 score of 5. She is very unwell and I urgently need your help. Is there anything else you would like me to do in the meantime?

Pneumonia in brief

1. What scoring system may be employed to determine the severity of pneumonia?

CURB-65

Confusion/ Abbreviated Mental Test Score ≤8	1
Urea >7 mmol/L	1
Respiratory Rate >30	1
Systolic BP <90 mmHg or Diastolic BP <60 mmHg	1
Age ≥65	1

Score:
- 0–1: low severity (risk of death 3 %) —> home treatment – with oral antiobiotics (if the patient has several co-morbidities, they can be managed in hospital with the same oral antibiotic).

- 2: moderate severity (risk of death 9 %) —> consider hospital admission and treatment with intravenous antibiotics, take blood cultures, send sputum for culture, urine for pneumococcal antigen (consider legionella and mycoplasma testing)

- 3–5: high severity (risk of death 15–40 %) —> hospital treatment with intravenous antibiotics, supportive care and investigations as above. May require critical care admission. Antibiotics will vary from hospital to hospital and you should follow your local hospital guidelines when deciding on the treatment.

2. How do you distinguish a community-acquired from a hospital-acquired pneumonia?
Hospital-acquired pneumonia is diagnosed in patients who develop a pneumonia ≥48– 72 hours after hospital admission, or in patients who have been in a healthcare setting over the past 3 months.

3. What are the common organisms responsible for community acquired pneumonia?
- Streptococcus pneumoniae (commonest)
- Haemophilus influenzae
- Staphylococcus aureus
- Mycoplasma pneumoniae

4. What are some of the complications of pneumonia?
- Respiratory failure
- Sepsis/septic shock
- Confusion
- Empyema

Case 3 – **Infective Exacerbation of COPD**

You are a Foundation Year 2 doctor working in A&E. Mr John Smith, who is a seventy-year old retired fisherman and a smoker with a forty pack-year history presents with an unrelenting productive cough. He is awaiting a review by the medical team when the nurse calls you for help, as his oxygen saturations have dropped from 90% to 83% and he has become more dyspnoeic.

Please conduct an A to E assessment of Mr Smith and commence the initial management.

Latest observations:
HR: 90; BP: 135/86; RR: 28; SaO$_2$: 83 % (room air); temp: 38.2 °C; U/O: NA

Danger
It is safe to approach Mr Smith.

Response
Mr Smith is alert and responsive, but is having difficulty completing full sentences.

Airway
Mr Smith is talking to you, so you are reassured that the airway is patent.

Breathing
Look – using accessory muscles, central cyanosis, producing green sputum
Feel – trachea is central; hyperexpanded chest, bilaterally reduced chest expansion
Listen – on auscultation there is poor air entry and widespread wheeze bilaterally
Measure – RR 28; SaO_2 83 % on room air
Treat – give oxygen through a Venturi mask to maintain SaO_2 between 88–92 %. Give salbutamol and ipratropium via a nebuliser and oral prednisolone
Reassess – his saturations are now 88 % on FiO_2 28% and RR is now 19

Further Investigations:
- ABG - demonstrates respiratory acidosis with type 2 respiratory failure
- Chest radiograph - lung hyperinflation
- Sputum microscopy and culture, urine antigens

Circulation
Look – appears clammy, some peripheral cyanosis
Feel – warm to touch, apex beat is not displaced
Listen – heart sounds normal
Measure – HR 90 bpm, regular; BP 135/86 CRT <2 seconds; temp: 38.2 °C; UO: NA
Treat – ensure IV antibiotics (as per hospital guidelines), IV fluids and paracetamol are given.

Further investigations:
- ECG (sinus rhythm)
- Bloods (FBC, U&E, LFTs, CRP)
- Blood cultures

Disability

AVPU – alert/GCS 15 (E4, V5, M6)
Capillary blood glucose – 5.7 mmol/L
Pupils – equal and reactive to light

Exposure

Fully expose the patient and perform a detailed secondary examination

Hand over to Dr Bullimore (Emergency Medicine SpR)

Situation: Good afternoon my name is _____ and I am the F2 in A&E. I would like to discuss Mr John Smith, who has suddenly deteriorated, dropped his saturations and became increasingly tachypnoeic.

Background: The patient was seen today with an infective exacerbation of COPD and was awaiting review by the medics. He is a retired fisherman with a forty pack-year history and a cough productive of green sputum.

Assessment: He is now stable after receiving oxygen (titrated to target saturations 88–92 %) and salbutamol and ipratropium nebulisers. His RR is now 19 breaths/minute after treatment, his saturations are 88 % on 28% oxygen delivered via a Venturi mask. His heart rate, BP, and CRT are normal, but he has a pyrexia of 38.2 °C. His ABG showed respiratory acidosis with type 2 respiratory failure. He is alert and his capillary blood glucose is normal.

Recommendation: I would like for you to come and review him to determine a further course of action. I will repeat his ABG in 30 minutes to reassess whether or not he requires non-invasive ventilation. Would you like me to do anything further?

COPD in brief

1. What is the underlying pathology of COPD?

The abnormality in COPD is chronic inflammation which affects the airways as well as the lung parenchyma, alveoli and blood vessels. This leads to remodelling and narrowing of the airways, proliferation of mucus secreting glands and goblet cells and finally changes in the vasculature leading to pulmonary hypertension. The main inflammatory cells involved include neutrophils, macrophages and leukocytes. There are two subtypes of COPD: emphysema and chronic bronchitis. In emphysema chronic inflammation results in elastin breakdown and loss of alveoli. In chronic bronchitis the inflammation leads to ciliary dysfunction, proliferation of goblet cells and increased mucus production.

2. What is the defining clinical feature of COPD?

Irreversible and progressive airflow limitation, formally diagnosed with spirometry (FEV_1/FVC <70 % of predicted)

3. What are the stages of COPD?

Stages of COPD are used to determine the severity of airflow obstruction and are based on spirometry readings. However, these correlate poorly with disease severity.

Stage	Forced Expiratory Volume	Management Recommendations
Stage I (mild)	FEV_1 80 % or greater of predicted	reduction of risk factors (influenza vaccine); short-acting bronchodilators
Stage II (moderate)	FEV_1 50–79 % of predicted	as for Stage I plus long-acting bronchodilator; cardiopulmonary rehabilitation
Stage III (severe)	FEV_1 30–49 % of predicted	as for Stages I and II plus inhaled glucocorticoids if repeated exacerbations
Stage IV (very severe)	FEV_1 <30 % of predicted or FEV_1 <50 % and chronic respiratory failure	as for Stages I – III plus long term oxygen (if meeting criteria); consideration of surgical options

4. In whom should long term oxygen therapy be considered?

- Stable individuals with severe symptoms and PaO_2 <7.3 kPa or oxygen saturations <88 % despite maximal medical therapy
- Individuals with PaO_2 of 7.3–8.0 kPa and with pulmonary hypertension, polycythaemia, peripheral oedema or nocturnal hypoxia

5. What are the complications of COPD?

- Recurrent exacerbations
- Chest infections
- Cor pulmonale
- Pneumothorax
- Respiratory failure
- Lung malignancy

Case 4 – **Acute Exacerbation of Asthma**

You are a Foundation Year 2 doctor working in the Emergency Department. A 20-year-old lady, Ms Shirley Jenner, presents with worsening shortness of breath, wheeze, and tightness in her chest. She has a past medical history of asthma and was last hospitalised with an acute exacerbation one year ago.

Please conduct an A to E assessment of Ms Jenner and commence the initial management.

Latest observations:
HR 120; BP 120/80; RR 30; SaO$_2$ 92 % (room air); temp 36.5 °C U/O: NA

Danger

It is safe to approach Ms Jenner.

Response

Ms Jenner is alert and responsive, but is unable to complete full sentences.

Airway

Look – no signs of airway obstruction or evidence of oedema
Feel – it is clear that she is breathing so no need to feel for movement of air
Listen – you are able to hear a wheeze from the end of the bed
Treat – adjust her position so that she is sitting upright

Breathing

Look – distressed, no evidence of cyanosis; using accessory muscles for respiration
Feel – the trachea is central; it is difficult to assess chest expansion
Listen – on auscultation there is poor air entry and widespread wheeze bilaterally
Measure – RR 30; SaO_2 92 % (room air)
Treat – give oxygen to maintain SaO_2 between 94–98 %; salbutamol and ipratropium nebulisers; prednisolone orally or intravenous hydrocortisone.
Reassess – her saturations rise to 95 % on 5L of oxygen and RR is now 22; she appears more comfortable and is no longer in respiratory distress. The air entry has improved, however a mild wheeze persists.

Further investigations:
- ABG - demonstrates type 1 respiratory failure with respiratory alkalosis and a potassium of 4.7 mmol/L
- Chest radiograph - no abnormalities detected
- Peak expiratory flow rate (compare to her baseline).

Circulation

Look – appears pale and clammy, no evidence of cyanosis
Feel – apex beat is not displaced, peripheries of normal temperature, normal skin turgor
Listen – heart sounds normal
Measure – HR 120 bpm, regular; BP 120/80; CRT <2 seconds; temp 36.5 °C
Treat – obtain IV access and consider further investigations

Further investigations:
- ECG monitoring - sinus tachycardia

Disability

AVPU – alert/GCS 15 (E4, V5, M6)
Capillary blood glucose – 5.9 mmol/L
Pupils – equal and reactive to light

Exposure

Fully expose the patient and perform a detailed secondary examination

Hand over to Dr Martin (Emergency Medicine SpR)

Situation – Good morning Dr Martin my name is _____ and I am the F2 in A&E. I would like to discuss Shirley Jenner who I suspect has an acute severe exacerbation of her asthma.

Background – Her past medical history includes asthma with a hospital admission one year ago.

Assessment – She has improved after administration of salbutamol and ipratropium nebulisers and I have given her oral steroids early on. But I am worried that she remains unwell. Her airway is clear at present. Her respiratory rate has improved from 30 to 22; her saturations are 95 % on 5 L and after nebulisers. The air entry has improved bilaterally but she remains wheezy. Her peak flow remains way below her baseline. Her HR, BP, and CRT are all within normal limits and she is apyrexial. She is alert at present and her blood capillary glucose was 5.9 mmol/L.

Recommendation – I would like for you to come and review her, as she remains tachypnoeic and wheezy and I feel she may require senior input. Is there anything you would like me to do until you are able to attend?

Asthma in brief

1. How is severity of an acute exacerbation of asthma classified?

Moderate Exacerbation	Acute Severe Asthma	Life-threatening Asthma
PEFR >50–75 % of predicted	PEFR 33–50 % of predicted	PEFR <33 % of predicted
no features of acute severe asthma	respiratory rate ≥25 breaths per minute	SpO_2 <92 %
	heart rate ≥110 beats per minute	PaO_2 <8 kPa
	inability to complete sentences in one breath	Normal or rising $PaCO_2$ (4.6– 6.0 kPa)
		Silent chest
		Drowsy or confused

PEFR – Peak Expiratory Flow Rate

2. How might the results of arterial blood gases change during the various stages of status asthmaticus?
- Stage one: hyperventilation —> normal pO_2 and low pCO_2
- Stage two: hyperventilation with hypoxaemia —> low pO_2 and low pCO_2
- Stage three: rate of ventilation begins to decrease as respiratory fatigue begins to set in —> low pO_2, normal pCO_2 (may require intubation)
- Stage four: respiratory muscles fail —> low pO_2 and high pCO_2

3. After administration of salbutamol and ipratropium nebulisers, the repeat ABG revealed a $PaCO_2$ of 4.6 kPA, what would be the next step?
- call for immediate senior assistance if you have not already done so
- give/repeat salbutamol via an oxygen-driven nebuliser
- consider back-to-back salbutamol nebulisers
- consider IV magnesium sulphate following a discussion with your seniors
- correct fluid and electrolytes, especially potassium, as salbutamol can lead to hypokalaemia
- repeat the ABG whenever there is a change in clinical state or when considering an alternation in management

4. What considerations should be made when preparing to discharge a patient who has been admitted with an acute exacerbation of asthma?
- if a patient has received nebulised beta 2 agonists prior to presentation, consider an extended observation period prior to discharge
- if PEFR <50 % of predicted at the time of presentation, prescribe prednisolone for five days
- ensure that the patient has adequate treatment supply of inhaled corticosteroid and beta 2 agonist and review inhaler technique
- arrange for follow-up with the GP within two weeks following discharge – including completing relevant paperwork
- refer to asthma liaison nurse or asthma clinic for consideration of stepping up regular treatment

Case 5 – **Pulmonary Embolism (PE)**

You are a Foundation Year 1 doctor on a general surgery ward. Mr Thomas James was admitted to hospital eight days ago for an emergency Hartmann's procedure due to perforation of a sigmoid diverticulum. He has been making a good recovery, but as you are about to end your shift, the nurse tells you that he has dropped his oxygen saturations and has become tachypnoeic.

Please conduct an A to E assessment of Mr James and commence the initial management.

Latest observations:
HR: 110; BP: 100/60; RR: 30; SaO$_2$: 86 % (room air); Temp: 36.0 °C; U/O: NA

Danger
It is safe to approach the patient

Response
Mr James is alert and sitting up in his bed

Airway
Mr James explains to you that he has suddenly started feeling short of breath, so you are reassured that the airway is patent

Breathing
Look – tachypnoeic, but is otherwise comfortable at rest
Feel – trachea is central and chest expansion is equal
Listen – good air entry bilaterally
Measure – RR 30, sats 86 % on room air
Treat – give oxygen to maintain SaO_2 between 94–98 %
Reassess – his saturations rise to 98 % on 15L of oxygen and RR is now 22

Further Investigations:
- ABG - type 1 respiratory failure with respiratory alkalosis
- Chest radiograph - no abnormalities

Circulation
Look – no evidence of sweating nor is he cyanosed; JVP is normal
Feel – he is tachycardic, but rhythm is regular; CRT <2 seconds
Listen – heart sounds normal
Measure – HR 110, regular; BP 100/60, temp 36.0 °C, U/O: not available
Treat – obtain IV access and consider further investigations

Further investigations:
- Bloods (clotting)
- d-Dimer unlikely to be helpful given the recent surgery
- ECG – sinus tachycardia
- Place patient on continuous cardiac monitoring
- Echocardiogram if trained operator available

Disability

AVPU – alert/GCS 15 (E4, V5, M6)
Capillary blood glucose – 5.5 mmol/L
Pupils – equal and reactive to light

Exposure

On full exposure, there is no evidence of bleeding from the wound, and the abdomen is soft and non-tender. The examination of the lower limb reveals a swollen left calf which is hot, firm and tender to palpation. Perform a Well's score assessment at this stage to determine the risk of a pulmonary embolus (see below).

Further investigate with an ultrasound (US) doppler scan and a CT pulmonary angiography (CTPA). Consider treatment with low molecular weight heparin if CTPA cannot be performed immediately following discussion with the surgical team.

Hand over to Mr Morrison (General Surgery SpR)

Situation – Good morning Mr Morrison my name is _____ and I am the F1 in General Surgery. I am calling regarding Mr Thomas James who I suspect has developed a pulmonary embolism.

Background – He underwent a Hartmann's procedure eight days ago which was uneventful.

Assessment – he has suddenly become tachypnoeic (RR 30) and hypoxic (saturations of 86 % on room air) an hour ago. He has a BP of 100/60 and HR of 110 bpm. I treated him with high-flow oxygen and his saturations improved to 98 % on 15 L and his RR came down to 22. Examination of the precordium was unremarkable and he had good air entry bilaterally.
Examination of the lower limbs revealed a swollen red left calf, which was tender to palpation and would be in keeping with a DVT. I have sent off routine bloods and have requested a chest x-ray. ECG revealed a sinus tachycardia with an S wave in lead I and Q wave and T wave inversion in lead III.

Recommendation – I suspect Mr James has a pulmonary embolus and I was hoping that you might be able to come and review this gentleman. In the meantime I will order an US scan of the lower limbs and a CTPA. Would you like me to commence treatment with low molecular weight heparin?

Pulmonary embolism in brief

1. What tool can be used to undertake a clinical risk assessment for pulmonary embolism?
Well's Score

Clinical Feature	Points
Signs/symptoms of DVT (leg swelling and pain on deep vein palpation)	3
PE most likely clinical diagnosis	3
HR >100	1.5
>3 days immobilisation or surgery in past 4 weeks	1.5
Previous DVT/PE	1.5
Haemoptysis	1
Malignancy (current treatment or treatment in past 6 months or palliative)	1

Score ≤4 is low risk: test for D-dimer
- if elevated —> CTPA
- if negative —> consider an alternative diagnosis

Score >4 is high risk: proceed to CTPA (cover with LMWH if scan cannot be performed immediately)

2. What are the treatment options for a pulmonary embolus?
Pulmonary embolus is usually managed with low molecular weight heparin according to local hospital policy. The patients are also commenced on warfarin or rivaroxaban depending on individual circumstances.

Massive pulmonary embolus, which leads to haemodynamic instability, may require thrombolysis with agents such as alteplase. If despite anticoagulation patients continue to get pulmonary emboli, then an inferior vena cava filter may be considered.

3. What are the absolute contraindications for thrombolysis of a pulmonary embolus?
- Haemorrhagic stroke or stroke of unknown origin at any time
- Ischaemic stroke in preceding six months
- Central nervous system injury
- Major trauma/head injury/surgery in the preceding three weeks
- Gastro-intestinal bleed within the past six months
- Known bleeding risk

4.What forms of anticoagulation are used in the treatment of a pulmonary embolus?
The guidelines for this vary greatly between individual hospitals. However, most hospitals will use either low molecular weight heparin or warfarin for specific time periods.

In addition to warfarin, rivaroxaban and apixaban (oral direct factor Xa inhibitors) are being used more frequently now in the treatment and prevention of pulmonary emboli. You should seek advice on their use from your hospital's haematology department.

However, it is important to note that rivaroxaban is contraindicated in active malignancy and renal failure with a creatinine clearance of less than 15. In these cases warfarin would be more suitable.

Cardiac Emergencies

Weiguang Loh

Cardiopulmonary Arrest	48
Hypertensive Crises	54
Aortic Dissection	58
Acute Heart Failure	62
Acute Coronary Syndrome	66
Atrial Fibrillation	70
Bradycardia and Heart Block	74
Cardiac Tamponade	78

Case 1 – **Cardiopulmonary Arrest**

You are a Foundation Year 1 doctor working on the acute medical unit. A nurse comes running towards you saying that Mr Dodds, an 83 year old patient, has suddenly stopped breathing while in his bed. She looks very distressed. Mr Dodds has a long history of coronary artery disease and has been admitted with acute kidney injury but is normally functionally independent. He was complaining of dizziness, chest pain and palpitations 10 minutes before the incident.

Please conduct an A to E assessment of Mr Dodds and commence the initial management.

Latest observations unavailable.

Danger
It is safe to approach the patient.

Response
Mr Dodds is unresponsive. It would be appropriate to shout for help at this stage.

Airway
Perform the head-tilt chin-lift procedure
Look – Nothing is seen obstructing the airway

Breathing
Look, feel and listen for any signs of life for a maximum of 10 seconds. One may also check the presence of any carotid pulse at the same time
Look – Absent chest movements. Patient appears cyanotic
Feel – No breaths felt, no carotid pulse felt
Listen – Absent breath sounds
Treat – CPR needs to be commenced immediately (unless a Do Not Attempt Resuscitation form has previously been issued)
Call the crash team

Commence cardio-pulmonary resuscitation. As per UK resuscitation guidelines, this involves repeated cycles of 30 chest compressions followed by 2 rescue breaths. Chest compressions are performed with placing a hand palm-down on the middle of the patient's sternum, the other hand palm-down on top, with fingers interlocking. The patient's chest should then be compressed as follows:
    Depth: 5 cm or 1/3 of the patients antero-posterior chest diameter.
    Rate: 100 – 120 compressions per minute

Rescue breaths should be performed via a bag-valve mask with high flow oxygen supply attached. The head-tilt chin-lift should be maintained by an assistant. Airway adjuncts may also be used. Each breath should be delivered over 1 second. Eventually, the patient will have to be intubated and a definite airway established. Once the patient has been intubated he can be ventilated with 10-12 breaths per minute.

The crash team now arrives. They hand the automated external defibrillator pads to you.

You should place the defibrillator pads on the patient and follow the instructions on the defibrillator, first turning it on and then assessing the patient's heart rhythm.

The patient's heart rhythm is the following, please proceed:
- Ventricular tachycardia (VT) OR
- Ventricular fibrillation (VF)

One should recognise that this is pulseless VT/VF and that this is a shockable rhythm as per Advanced Life Support Guidelines.

Perform one shock at 150 – 200 Joules biphasic and immediately resume chest compressions for another 2-minute cycle of 30 compressions to 2 breaths.

Reassess and if there are still no signs of life, perform another shock and repeat the cycle of 30:2.

Give adrenaline 1mg IV (1:10 000) in a prefilled syringe and amiodarone 300 mg IV after the third shock.

Give adrenaline 1mg IV (1:10 000) every 3 – 5 minutes thereafter.

Don't forget to check for the reversible causes of a cardiac arrest.
4 Hs:
- Hypoxia
- Hypovolaemia
- Hypothermia
- Hyperkalaemia/hypokalaemia/hypocalcaemia

4 Ts:
- Tension pneumothorax
- Tamponade
- Toxins
- Thromboembolism

The patient suddenly has a return of spontaneous circulation

You should now reassess the patient using the ABCDE approach and refer the patient to the intensive care unit.

Hand over the patient to Dr Shivani (Critical Care SpR)

Situation – My name is Dr_____ and I am an F1 in acute medicine. This patient is Mr Dodds, an 83 year old gentleman who suddenly went into a cardiopulmonary arrest. There was return of spontaneous circulation after 5 cycles of CPR.

Background – Mr Dodds has a long history of coronary artery disease and has been admitted under the medics with AKI.

Assessment – On initial assessment, Mr Dodds was unresponsive and appeared cyanosed. No breaths were seen, felt or heard for 10 seconds. The carotid pulse was also absent. Hence CPR was started and the crash team called. The ECG trace showed pulseless VT/VF. The Advanced Life Support algorithm was commenced and the defibrillator applied. Adrenaline and amiodarone were also given and the patient was intubated. After 5 cycles of CPR there was return of spontaneous circulation.

Recommendation – The patient requires critical care admission, and close monitoring, as well as further investigations for the underlying cause.

Cardiopulmonary arrest (ALS) in brief:

It is important to memorize the ALS protocol as the minutiae of the algorithm may be confusing (see Figure 1). It is also vital to be able to recognise the two shockable rhythms and identify them quickly on the ECG.

1. What is the management of the shockable rhythms?
The management of the shockable rhythms, namely VF and pulseless VT, is via non-synchronised DC cardioversion. Patients require a shock every 2 minutes alternating with cycles of 30 compressions to 2 breaths. Adrenaline 1 mg IV (1:10 000) and amiodarone 300 mg IV stat are given after the third shock and further adrenaline injections are given every 3 – 5 minutes thereafter (ie. every 2 subsequent shocks).

2. What is the management of the non-shockable rhythms?
The management of the non-shockable rhythms, namely pulseless electrical activity and asystole, require continuation of CPR in 30:2 ratio. Adrenaline 1 mg IV (1:10 000) is given immediately and every 3 – 5 minutes thereafter.

Figure 1. Advanced Life Support (ALS) Algorithm (Adapted from the Resuscitation Council UK)

If patient unresponsive, call for help and proceed as per BLS protocol *see Figure 2*

⬇

If patient has not yet recovered by the time the crash team arrives, follow the ALS protocol by assessing the patient's rhythm

⬇

Shockable rhythm

⬇

Shock the patient once (150 – 200 Joules biphasic) and continue 2 minute CPR cycles of 30 chest compressions to 2 rescue breaths.

⬇

Keep assessing for signs of life and reversible causes while repeating the cycles of 1 shock followed by 2 minutes of CPR

⬇

Give adrenaline 1 mg IV 1:10,000 and amiodarone 300 mg IV after third shock

⬇

Give adrenaline 1 mg IV 1:10,000 every 3 – 5 minutes thereafter (ie. after every other shock)

If unshockable rhythm (ie. PEA or asystole)

⬇

Do NOT shock the patient. Give adrenaline 1 mg IV 1:10,000 and commence CPR

⬇

Keep assessing for signs of life and reversible causes while performing CPR and repeat adrenaline 1mg IV 1:10,000 every 3 – 5 minutes thereafter

⬇

If signs of life appear begin ABCDE assessment

Figure 2. Basic Life Support Algorithm (Adapted from the Resuscitation Council UK)

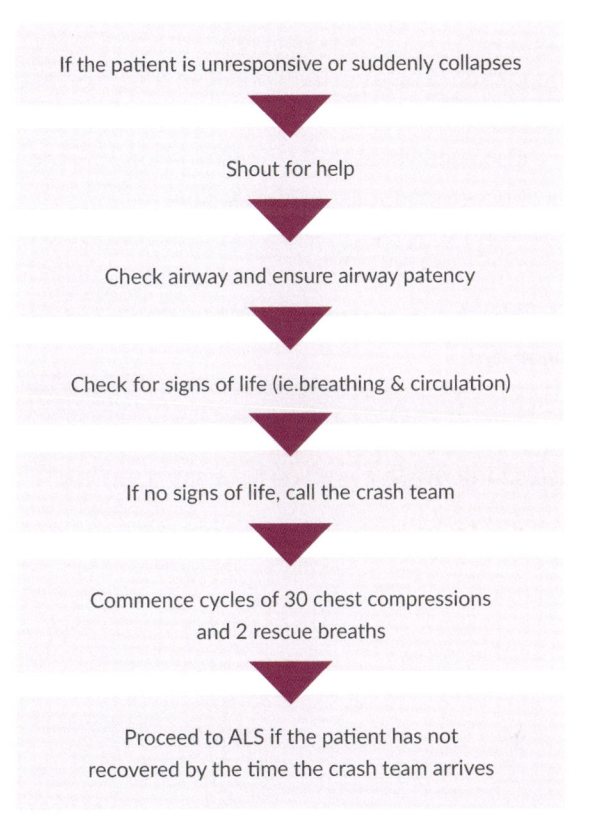

If the patient is unresponsive or suddenly collapses

⬇

Shout for help

⬇

Check airway and ensure airway patency

⬇

Check for signs of life (ie. breathing & circulation)

⬇

If no signs of life, call the crash team

⬇

Commence cycles of 30 chest compressions and 2 rescue breaths

⬇

Proceed to ALS if the patient has not recovered by the time the crash team arrives

Case 2 – **Hypertensive Crises**

You are a Foundation Year 2 doctor working in the Emergency Department. A 40 year old lady, Mrs Davis, presents complaining of shortness of breath, a headache, nausea and vomiting. Her husband informs you that Mrs Davis has a history of poorly controlled hypertension.

Please conduct an A to E assessment of Mrs Davis and commence the initial management.

Latest observations:
HR: 140 BP: 220/134 RR: 29 SaO$_2$: 92 % (RA) Temp: 36.9 °C UO: NA

Danger
It is safe to approach the patient.

Response
Mrs Davis is responsive, but is groaning in pain and appears confused. Ask for senior help at this stage.

Airway
Look – Nothing seen obstructing the airway
Feel – Trachea not deviated
Listen – Rapid laboured breathing
Treat – The patient is maintaining her airway, no treatment necessary

Breathing
Look – Distressed, rapid laboured breathing
Feel – Chest expansion and percussion normal
Listen – Bibasal crepitations
Measure – RR: 29, SaO_2 92 % on room air
Treat – As the patient is tachypnoeic and hypoxic, supplemental oxygen should be administered
Reassess – RR: 27, SaO_2 95 %, patient is still in distress

Further investigations:
- ABG - type 1 respiratory failure
- Chest X-ray - pulmonary oedema

Circulation
Look – Distressed, JVP raised
Feel – Sweaty, apex beat thrusting but not displaced
Listen – Quiet heart sounds
Measure – HR: 140, Regular, BP: 220/134 (similar in both arms), Temp: 36.9 °C
Treat – Consider invasive blood pressure monitoring i.e. an arterial line. Intravenous boluses of labetolol or a labetolol infusion can then be used to lower the BP. This should only be initiated under senior supervision
Reassess – HR 128, BP 170/130, Temp: 36.9 °C

Further investigations:
- ECG - sinus tachycardia, left axis deviation, tall R waves in lateral leads
- Bloods (FBC, U&E, LFT, TFT)
- Urine dipstick

It is important to recognise a hypertensive crisis in this patient. The patient has signs of hypertensive encephalopathy as evidenced by the headache, nausea and vomiting. She may also have papilloedema on fundoscopy and visual changes. A controlled reduction in her blood pressure will alleviate her symptoms and is normally done with intravenous labetalol. However, in this case you may wish to call for senior help first. The patient also requires admission to the high dependency unit for monitoring.

Disability

AVPU – Responsive to pain/ GCS 9 (E1V3M5)
Blood glucose – 5.5 mmol/L
Pupils – Equal and reactive to light. There are papilloedema and retinal haemorrhages on fundoscopy (hypertensive retinopathy grade IV).

Exposure

Fully expose the patient and perform a detailed head-to-toe examination. On full exposure, there is no evidence of bleeding or rashes and the abdomen is soft and non-tender. No localising neurological signs on the neurological examination.

Hand over the patient to Dr Patel (Critical Care SpR)

Situation – My name is Dr_____ and I am the FY2 working in A&E. I have been called to assess Mrs Davis, who presents with a hypertensive crisis.

Background – She is a 40 year old woman who was admitted complaining of severe shortness of breath, headaches, nausea and vomiting. Mrs Davis has a history of uncontrolled hypertension.

Assessment – On initial assessment Mrs Davis was only responsive to voice. Her observations were HR: 140 BP: 220/134 RR: 29 SaO_2: 92 % Temp: 36.9 °C. She was dyspnoeic, had a thrusting apex beat and a raised JVP. I suspected a hypertensive crisis and have given her high flow oxygen and inserted 2 intravenous cannulae.

Recommendation – I would like you to review this patient, and consider invasive blood pressure monitoring and commencing intravenous labetalol for a controlled reduction in her blood pressure.

Hypertensive crises in brief:

1. What is a hypertensive crisis?
Severe hypertension is when a patient has a systolic blood pressure of 180 mmHg or higher, or a diastolic blood pressure of 110 mmHg or higher, or both (figures may vary depending on classification). If not appropriately managed, this can lead to a hypertensive crisis, due to damage to blood vessels and resultant cardiac dysfunction. There are 2 main types of hypertensive crises:
1. Hypertensive urgency, with no obvious end-organ damage, or
2. Malignant/Accelerated hypertension, whereby there is end-organ damage.

Examples of end-organ damage include: cardiovascular dysfunction, pulmonary oedema, renal failure, papilloedema or, as in this patient, encephalopathy. The difference in management of the two types being that hypertensive urgency can be treated over 1 – 2 days while malignant/accelerated hypertension requires immediate treatment.

2. What is the management of a hypertensive crisis?
The management of a hypertensive crisis is usually supervised by a senior cardiology physician as there is a wide range of possible pharmacological treatments available, with varying mechanisms of action. Sympathetic blockers such as labetalol or phentolamine, vasodilators such as hydralazine, nitroglyceride or nitroprusside or diuretics may be used in different scenarios. Many centers use modified release nifedipine which is a calcium channel blocker.

3. What other investigations should be performed?
The underlying cause of hypertension should be investigated in young patients or in severe uncontrollable hypertension. The investigations should include: urinary protein-creatinine ratio, 24-hour urinary metanephrines, urinary free cortisol, dexamethasone suppression test, renin-aldosterone levels and imaging of the renal arteries. Other risk factors such as diabetes and hyperlipidaemia should also be looked for in these patients.

4. What are the causes of hypertension?
Primary essential hypertension is the commonest cause worldwide but the underlying cause remains unknown.

Secondary hypertension can occur as a result of:
- Intrinsic renal disease – glomerulonephritides, polycystic kidney disease
- Renal vascular disease – renal artery stenosis due to atherosclerosis or fibrodysplasia
- Connective tissue disease – scleroderma
- Endocrine disease – acromegaly, phaechromocytoma, Cushing's and Conn's syndromes
- Drugs – steroids, oral contraceptive pill, monoamine oxidase inhibitors, sympathomimetics

Case 3 – **Aortic Dissection**

You are a Foundation Year 2 doctor working in A&E. Mr Reed, a 40 year old gentleman, presents complaining of a sudden onset sharp, tearing chest pain radiating to his back. You notice that he looks marfanoid and his wife informs you that he has a history of hypertension. Mr Reed also complains of paraesthesia in his left arm.

Please conduct an A to E assessment of Mr Reed and commence the initial management.

Latest observations:
HR: 110. BP: Variable in both arms: Right 160/90; Left 130/70. RR: 27 SaO_2: 98 % (RA) Temp 36.9 °C UO: NA

Danger

It is safe to approach Mr Reed.

Response

Mr Reed is alert but in distress.

Airway

Look – Nothing is seen obstructing the airway
Feel – Trachea is not deviated
Listen – Patient appears slightly dyspnoeic
Treat – The patient is maintaining his airway, no treatment is necessary

Breathing

Look – Distressed
Feel – Chest expansion and percussion normal
Listen – Bilateral air entry present
Measure – RR 27, SaO_2 98 % (RA)
Treat – No treatment necessary at this point

Further investigations:
- Chest X-ray - widened mediastinum

Circulation

Look – Peripheral pallor, JVP not visible
Feel – Cold peripheries, CRT in the left hand is 7 seconds, radial-radial pulse delay
Listen – Early diastolic murmur
Measure – HR: 110, BP: variable in both arms: Right 160/90, Left 130/70, Temp 36.9 °C, UO: NA
Treat – obtain intravenous access and titrate intravenous analgesia (i.e. morphine) to pain. This patient's blood pressure needs to be lowered cautiously (with intravenous labetalol or nitroprusside) by an experienced clinician. This will require invasive blood pressure monitoring (e.g. an arterial line) within a high dependency setting. Therefore ask for senior help early on. A urinary catheter should also be inserted for accurate fluid balance monitoring.

The classic history of a sudden onset sharp tearing chest pain radiating to the back coupled with variable pulse rate and blood pressure in both arms should prompt you to think that this is likely an aortic dissection.

The patient should be closely monitored within a high dependency setting. The management of an aortic dissection generally involves reducing the patient's blood pressure and heart rate using nitroprusside, beta blockers or calcium channel blockers. The patient should then be discussed with your seniors and a surgical or an endovascular intervention planned.

Further investigations:
- ECG
- Further cardiac imaging – transthoracic echocardiography; CT angiography is used to confirm the diagnosis and identify the extent and location of the dissection
- Bloods (FBC, U&E, LFT, Coagulation)
- Crossmatch 6 units of red blood cells, fresh frozen plasma and platelets

Disability

AVPU – Patient is alert
Blood glucose – 5.5 mmol/L
Pupils – Equal and reactive to light

Exposure

Fully expose the patient and perform a detailed head to toe examination. On full exposure, there is no evidence of bleeding or rashes and the abdomen is soft and non-tender. Normal full neurological examination.

Hand over the patient to Dr Patel (Critical Care SpR)

Situation – My name is Dr_____ and I am the FY2 in A&E. I have been called to assess Mr Reed, a 40 year old gentleman with an aortic dissection.

Background – Mr Reed has a history of hypertension and presented complaining of a sudden onset sharp, tearing chest pain radiating to his back with paraesthesia in his left arm.

Assessment – On initial assessment the patient was alert but in severe distress. His observations were HR: 110; BP is variable in the arms: right 160/90, left 130/70; RR: 27; SaO2: 98 %; Temp 36.9 °C. He had cool peripheries, a CRT of 7 seconds in the left arm, radial-radial pulse delay and evidence of aortic regurgitation on a transthoracic echocardiogram. A CT angiography demonstrated an ascending aortic dissection. I have obtained intravenous access and crossmatched 6 units of blood, FFP and platelets.

Recommendation – I would like you to review this patient and consider invasive BP monitoring and intravenous BP lowering therapy. In the meantime I will discuss the case with a cardiothoracic unit regarding a surgical or endovascular intervention.

Aortic dissection in brief:

1. What is an aortic dissection?
Aortic dissection occurs when there is a tear in the intima layer of the aorta. Blood, being forced through the aorta under high pressure, ends up entering the tear, further separating the intima layer from the adventitia and creating a false lumen. As more blood enters, the false lumen enlarges and may occlude smaller vessels such as the coronary, spinal, carotid, brachiocephalic and subclavian arteries.

2. What is the management of an aortic dissection?
The management of an aortic dissection involves invasive monitoring and reduction in the patient's blood pressure and heart rate simultaneously with nitroprusside and beta blockers such as labetalol. Opioid analgesia is given for the severe pain and also helps to lower the blood pressure and heart rate. A surgical or endovascular intervention is offered depending on the patient and the type of the dissection. This is done to prevent any further complications such as aortic rupture.

3. What are the risk factors of an aortic dissection?
Risk factors leading to an aortic dissection include connective tissue diseases such as Marfan's or Ehlers-Danlos syndromes, hypertension, smoking, hyperlipidaemia, atherosclerosis, trauma or vessel degeneration. An aortic aneurysm may also lead to aortic dissection. Hence, those with an inherited cause, which is likely to predispose them to dissections, and those with a known aortic aneurysm should have pristine blood pressure control and regular echocardiograms.

Case 4 – **Acute Heart Failure**

You are a Foundation Year 2 doctor working in the Emergency Department. Mrs Richardson, a 75 year old lady is brought into A&E severely short of breath and feeling generally unwell. She has a known history of myocardial infarction and left ventricular dysfunction.

Please conduct an A to E assessment of Mrs Richardson and commence the initial management.

Latest observations:
HR: 110 BP: 150/100. RR: 27 SaO$_2$: 89 % (RA) Temp 36.9 °C UO: NA

Danger
It is safe to approach Mrs Richardson

Response
Mrs Richardson is alert, but too short of breath to talk to you

Airway
Look – Nothing is obstructing the airway; the patient appears moderately dyspnoeic
Feel – Trachea is not deviated
Listen – No added breath sounds
Treat – The patient is maintaining her airway, no treatment is necessary

Breathing
Look – Moderately dyspnoeic, pale, clammy
Feel – Chest expansion and percussion normal
Listen – Bilateral air entry with bibasal crackles
Measure – RR 27, SaO_2 89 % on room air
Treat – High flow oxygen (15 L via a non-rebreath mask) should be given
Reassess – Patient is still dyspnoeic but SaO_2 is now 94 %

Further investigations:
- ABG - type 1 respiratory failure (repeat after starting oxygen therapy)
- Chest X-ray - pulmonary oedema, bilateral pleural effusions, Kerley-B lines

Circulation
Look – Pale, clammy, JVP 6 cm, bilateral pitting ankle swelling up to the knees
Feel – Cool peripheries, apex beat displaced to the left, CRT 3 seconds
Listen – Third heart sound present, right-sided heave
Measure - HR: 110 Regular. BP: 150/100 Temp 36.9 °C
Treat – sit the patient upright, obtain intravenous access. Give IV furosemide 40 – 80 mg, nitrates and morphine. Give low molecular weight heparin for thromboprophylaxis. Insert a urinary catheter for fluid balance monitoring
Reassess – HR: 85. BP 100/70. Patient no longer feels breathless

Further investigations:
- ECG - left axis deviation with left ventricular hypertrophy
- Daily weights to monitor fluid balance
- Echocardiogram - left ventricular dysfunction with a reduced ejection fraction
- Bloods (FBC, U&E, LFT, TFT, BNP, troponin)

> The presence of a raised JVP, bilateral ankle oedema, a third heart sound and bibasal crackles in a patient with severe dyspnoea suggests a diagnosis of congestive heart failure with pulmonary oedema. You should discuss the patient with your seniors.

Disability

AVPU – Patient is alert and fully responsive
Blood glucose – 6.0 mmol/L
Pupils – Equal and reactive to light

Exposure

Fully expose the patient and perform a detailed head to toe examination. Bilateral pitting ankle oedema up to the knees and sacral oedema is noted.

Hand over the patient to Dr Patel (Medical SpR)

Situation – My name is Dr_____ and I am the FY2 in A&E. I have seen Mrs Richardson, who has come in with acute congestive heart failure.

Background – Mrs Richardson has a history of myocardial infarcts and left ventricular dysfunction. She has come in complaining of difficulty breathing at rest.

Assessment – She was unable to talk because of the shortness of breath and her observations were HR: 110. BP: 150/100. RR: 27 SaO_2: 89 % (RA) Temp 36.9 °C. She was pale, clammy, had a JVP of 6 cm and bilateral pitting oedema up to her knees. Her apex beat was displaced and a right sided heave was noted with a third heart sound. She had bibasal crackles in her lungs. I suspected a diagnosis of acute congestive heart failure with pulmonary oedema and commenced high flow oxygen and sat her upright. I have obtained IV access and administered furosemide, nitrates and morphine. Her condition has now improved and she is feeling better.

Recommendation – I would like you to review this patient and consider further investigations and management of her heart failure.

Acute heart failure in brief:

1. What is heart failure?
Heart failure is a clinical syndrome when the heart fails to pump blood efficiently through the body as a result of reduced cardiac output, leading to tissue hypoperfusion, increased pulmonary pressure and tissue congestion. The diagnosis requires the presence of typical symptoms, signs and evidence of a structural or functional abnormality of the heart. Typical symptoms and signs of right sided heart failure include fatigue, pitting oedema, raised JVP and ascites. Those of left sided heart failure include exertional breathlessness, orthopnoea, paroxysmal nocturnal dyspnoea, nocturnal cough, cardiac wheeze and bibasal crackles.

2. What are the common causes of acute heart failure?

- Decompensation of pre-existing chronic heart failure
- Acute coronary syndrome
- Severe hypertension
- Valvular heart disease
- Myocarditis
- Cardiac tamponade
- Fluid overload (renal failure)

3. What immediate investigations can be performed in a patient with suspected acute heart failure?
Investigations include: an ECG to look for evidence of any arrhythmias, ischaemic changes and conduction defects; chest x-ray to look for evidence of heart failure (alveolar oedema, Kerley B lines, cardiomegaly, dilated upper lobe vessels, pleural effusion), echocardiogram to look for structural abnormalities and to measure ejection fraction to assess severity and brain natriuretic peptide (BNP) . A distinction between systolic and diastolic (preserved ejection fraction) heart failure may be made following an echocardiogram and aid further management.

4. What is the management of acute left ventricular heart failure?
The immediate management of acute heart failure involves sitting the patient upright to decrease venous return to the heart and subsequently offering loop diuretics. Vasodilators such as nitrates and opiates may be considered. Continuous Positive Airway Pressure (CPAP) ventilation may be used if the patient deteriorates. Once the patient is stable, further medical therapy with ACE inhibitors, beta-blockers, angiotensin-receptor blockers and spironolactone should be considered. Thromboprophylaxis should also be given.

Case 5 – **Acute Coronary Syndrome**

You are a Foundation Year 2 doctor working in the Emergency Department. Mr Ryan, a 55 year old gentleman comes into A&E complaining of severe crushing central chest pain radiating to his left arm. He has a past medical history of coronary artery disease, hypertension and increased cholesterol.

Please conduct an A to E assessment of Mr Ryan and commence the initial management.

Latest observations:
HR: 110 BP: 108/72 RR: 24 SaO_2: 91 % (RA), Temp 36.9 °C UO: NA

Danger
It is safe to approach Mr Ryan

Response
Mr Ryan is alert and fully responsive

Airway
Look – Nothing is seen obstructing the airway
Feel – Trachea is not deviated
Listen – No abnormal breath sounds
Treat – The patient is maintaining his airway, no treatment is necessary

Breathing
Look – Moderately dyspnoeic, pale, clammy
Feel – Chest expansion and percussion normal
Listen – Bilateral air entry
Measure – RR 24, SaO$_2$ 91 % (RA)
Treat – Oxygen should be offered
Reassess – Patient is still dyspnoeic but SaO$_2$ is now 96 %

Further investigations:
- ABG - before and after the initiation of oxygen therapy
- Chest X-ray

Circulation
Look – Pale, clammy, distressed and in severe pain, JVP not raised, no ankle swelling
Feel – Cool peripheries, apex beat not displaced
Listen – Heart sounds normal
Measure - HR: 110 BP: 108/72, Temp 36.9 °C, CRT 3 seconds
Treat – Obtain IV access. Give "MONA" – Morphine and an anti-emetic, oxygen , glyceril-tri-nitrate (GTN) and aspirin. Place patient on continuous cardiac monitoring. Discuss patient with a cardiologist with regards to further management.
Reassess – HR: 105 BP 105/71, Temp 36.9 °C

Further investigations:
- ECG - elevated ST segment over leads II, III and aVF
- Bloods (FBC, U&E, LFT, blood glucose, lipid profile, coagulation)
- Tropinin - raised (will need to be repeated to look at the trend)

Box 1.

You should refer to your local hospital guidelines on the treatment of acute coronary syndrome. Since this patient has an ST-segment elevated myocardial infarction, he should be discussed with the on-call cardiologist. This patient may benefit from restoration of coronary perfusion either with a primary percutaneous coronary intervention (PCI) or thrombolysis if the former is not available. All patients who present with an acute STEMI should undergo PCI as soon as possible. If PCI is unavailable then these patients should be thrombolysed with tissue plasminogen activators such as alteplase or reteplase. Patients undergoing PCI should also receive anticoagulation with agents such as bivalirudin (reversible direct thrombin inhibitor) or enoxaparin. Glycoprotein IIb/IIIa inhibitors such as abciximab or tirofiban can also be used. If PCI and thrombolysis are not available, then fondaparinux, enoxaparin or unfractioned heparin may be used.

Disability

AVPU – Patient alert and fully responsive/GCS15
Blood glucose – 5.8 mmol/L
Pupils – Equal and reactive to light

Exposure

Fully expose the patient and perform a detailed head to toe examination. On full exposure, there is no evidence of bleeding or rashes and the abdomen is soft and non-tender.

Hand over the patient to Dr Patel (Cardiology SpR)

Situation – My name is Dr_____ and I am the FY2 in A&E. I have just seen Mr Ryan who I suspect is having an inferior MI.

Background – Mr Ryan has multiple risk factors for ischaemic heart disease.

Assessment – His latest observations are HR: 105 BP: 105/71 RR: 24 SaO$_2$: 96 % (RA), Temp 36.9 °C. He was pale, clammy and in distress with severe pain. He had cool peripheries. His JVP was not raised and no ankle swelling was noted. Investigations revealed an elevated ST-segment over leads II, III and aVF with raised troponins. He has received morphine, high flow oxygen, GTN, aspirin and clopidogrel.

Recommendation – I would like you to review this patient with regards to performing a percutaneous coronary intervention. Would you like me to give him anticoagulation prior to PCI, and if so with which agent?

Acute coronary syndromes in brief:

1. What is an acute coronary syndrome?
Acute coronary syndrome, or ACS, is a cluster of acute myocardial ischaemic states, all of which usually present with chest pain or discomfort which commonly radiates to the left arm (or both), neck or jaw. There are 3 main types, namely ST-elevation myocardial infarction (STEMI), non-ST-elevation myocardial infarction (NSTEMI) and unstable angina. An ECG helps to differentiate a STEMI from an NSTEMI, while a raised troponin helps to differentiate angina from a myocardial infarction. The difference between stable and unstable angina is that in stable angina, the pain is usually preceded by predictable factors such as exertion whilst in unstable angina, the pain may even occur at rest without a known triggering factor.

2. What are the management options for the different types of acute coronary syndromes?
The management of unstable angina and NSTEMI are similar, with morphine, oxygen, nitrates and aspirin administered. Anticoagulation should be given and the Global Registry of Acute Cardiac Events (GRACE) risk score measured to predict the 6-month mortality. A GRACE score of more than 1.5 % requires clopidogrel or ticagrelor added onto the drug regime and a GRACE score of more than 3% requires a coronary angiography and possible percutaneous coronary intervention as soon as possible.

The management of STEMI involves morphine, oxygen, nitrates, aspirin and clopidogrel (once in the PCI lab). A coronary angiography and percutaneous coronary intervention should be performed as soon as possible, and these patients will require anticoagulation. Thrombolysis with alteplase may be used if PCI is unavailable (See Box 1).

Case 6 – **Atrial Fibrillation**

You are a Foundation Year 2 doctor working in the Emergency Department. Mrs Craig, a 73 year old lady, is rushed into A&E following a sudden collapse at home. On arrival, she is drowsy and breathless. Her carer mentions that she was complaining of palpitations just before the collapse.

Please conduct an A to E assessment of Mrs Craig and commence the initial management.

Latest observations:
HR: 160 BP: 89/60. RR: 32 SaO$_2$: 84 % (RA) Temp 36.9 °C UO: NA

Danger

It is safe to approach Mrs Craig.

Response

Mrs Craig is drowsy and responsive to pain. It would be appropriate to call for help.

Airway

Look – Nothing is seen obstructing the airway
Feel – Trachea is not deviated
Listen – Patient appears dyspnoeic
Treat – The patient is maintaining her airway, no treatment is necessary

Breathing

Look – Dyspnoeic, pale, clammy
Feel – Chest expansion and percussion normal
Listen – Bilateral air entry present. Mild bibasal crackles present
Measure – RR 32, SaO_2 84 % (RA)
Treat – High flow oxygen (15L via a non-rebreathe mask) should be offered
Reassess – The SaO_2 improves to 100 %

Further investigations:
- ABG - before and after oxygen therapy
- Chest X-ray

Circulation

Look – Pale, clammy, JVP 6cm, bilateral pitting oedema to the mid-calf observed
Feel – Irregularly irregular pulse, cool peripheries, CRT 3s, apex not displaced
Listen – Normal but irregular heart sounds
Measure - HR: 160 irregularly irregular, BP: 89/60, Temp 36.9 °C, UO: NA
Treat – Obtain IV access. The irregularly irregular tachyarrhythmia is suggestive of atrial fibrillation and in a haemodynamically unstable patient should prompt immediate treatment with synchronised DC cardioversion. Anticoagulation should be offered, but must not delay DC cardioversion. The patient should also be catheterised for careful fluid balance monitoring and should be placed on a cardiac monitor

Further investigations:
- ECG - shows an irregularly irregular tachyarrhythmia with absent P waves
- Bloods (FBC, U&E, LFT, TFT, troponin, calcium, magnesium, phosphate)
- Urgent echocardiogram to look for the underlying cause

Disability

AVPU – responds to pain/GCS 9 (E2, V2, M5)
Blood glucose – 5.8 mmol/L
Pupils – Equal and reactive to light

Exposure

Fully expose the patient and perform a detailed head to toe examination. On full exposure, there is no evidence of bleeding or rashes and the abdomen is soft and non-tender.

Hand over the patient to Dr Patel (Emergency Medicine SpR)

Situation – My name is Dr_____ and I am the FY2 in A&E. I have just seen Mrs Craig who presented with fast atrial fibrillation and haemodynamic instability.

Background – Mrs Craig was complaining of palpitations and chest pain just before she collapsed at home.

Assessment – Her observations were HR: 160 irregularly irregular. BP: 89/60. RR: 32 SaO_2: 84 % (RA) Temp 36.9 °C. She was dyspnoeic, pale, clammy with bibasal crackles and bilateral pitting oedema. CRT was 3 seconds and JVP was raised at 6cm. Her ECG showed an irregularly irregular tachyarrhythmia with absent P waves, confirming a diagnosis of atrial fibrillation.
I have given her high flow oxygen and inserted two IV cannulae into her arms thus far.

Recommendation – I would like you to review this patient with regards to performing an immediate synchronised DC cardioversion. I will also fast bleep the on call anaesthetist.

Atrial fibrillation in brief:

1. What is atrial fibrillation?
Atrial fibrillation (AF) is a common cardiac arrhythmia and is characterised by its irregularly irregular pulse with absent P waves on the ECG. The irregular contractions lead to a reduction in ventricular filling and hence a decrease in cardiac output. There is also an increased risk of thrombus formation leading to thrombo-embolic events, due to the stagnation of blood in the heart. There are many types of AF, namely acute AF (onset within the last 48 hours), paroxysmal AF (lasting up to 7 days), persistent AF (lasting more than 7 days), and permanent AF (lasting more than a year).

2. What is the management of atrial fibrillation?
The management depends on the type of AF, and whether the patient is haemodynamically compromised or not. Haemodynamically compromised patients, such as those with fast AF, heart failure as a result of the AF, hypotension or those with reduced conscious levels, require emergency electrical synchronised DC cardioversion. Low molecular weight heparin should be offered as anticoagulation.

The management of non-compromising AF involves either rate or rhythm control of the arrhythmia. Rate control includes giving either beta blockers, calcium channel blockers or digoxin. In rhythm control, electrical cardioversion, beta blockers flecainide or amiodarone may be used depending on the circumstances.

It is also important to evaluate the risk of ischaemic stroke (various scoring systems are available) in patients with atrial fibrillation and consider anticoagulation therapy with either warfarin or other newer anticoagulation drugs such as apixaban.

Any underlying triggers of AF such as infection, hyperthyroidism, conduction or cardiac structural abnormalities should be addressed.

There are multiple other tachyarrhythmias, which require specific treatment. However, as a general rule any tachyarrhythmia that is causing severe chest pain, reduced consciousness level, heart failure or haemodynamic compromise will require immediate cardioversion and senior input.

Case 7 – **Bradycardia and Heart Block**

You are a Foundation Year 2 doctor working in the Emergency Department. Mr Rhodes, a 75 year old gentleman, comes in with difficulty breathing, fatigue, dizziness and feeling generally unwell. He is currently not in any pain. He has a known history of ischaemic heart disease and normally takes atenolol. His GP recently started him on verapamil. He is unable to give any further details. .

Please conduct an A to E assessment of Mr Rhodes and commence the initial management.

Latest observations:
HR: 30 BP: 90/60. RR: 32 SaO$_2$ 90 % (RA) Temp 36.9 °C UO: NA

Danger

It is safe to approach Mr Rhodes.

Response

Mr Rhodes is drowsy. It would be appropriate to call for senior help at this stage.

Airway

Look – Nothing is seen obstructing the airway
Feel – Trachea is not deviated
Listen – No added breath sounds
Treat – The patient is maintaining his airway, no treatment is necessary

Breathing

Look – Severely dyspnoeic, pale, clammy
Feel – Chest expansion and percussion normal
Listen – Bilateral lower lung zone crackles
Measure – RR 32, SaO_2 90 % (RA)
Treat – High flow oxygen (15 L via a non-rebreathe mask) should be offered
Reassess – SaO_2 improves to 100 %

Further investigations:
- ABG - type 1 respiratory failure
- Chest X-ray - demonstrates mild pulmonary oedema

Circulation

Look – Pale, clammy, peripheral cyanosis, JVP 6cm
Feel – Cool peripheries, apex beat not displaced, CRT 4 seconds
Listen – normal but slow heart sounds
Measure - HR: 30 regular with every 5th beat absent. BP: 90/60 Temp 36.9 °C

Further investigations:
- ECG - shows complete discordance of P-waves and QRS complexes with no ischaemic changes
- Bloods (FBC, U&E, LFT, TFT, calcium, magnesium, phosphate, troponin)

Treat – The diagnosis of a third degree heart block should be made. Intravenous access should be obtained and the bradycardia should be managed with intravenous atropine. You should ask for a cardiology review.
Reassess – HR: 46 BP 100/70, Temp 36.9 °C

Disability

AVPU – Patient is responsive to voice/GCS 13 (E3V4M6)
Blood glucose – 5.8 mmol/L
Pupils – Equal and reactive to light

Exposure

Fully expose the patient and perform a detailed head to toe examination. On full exposure, there is no evidence of bleeding, rashes and the abdomen is soft and non-tender

Hand over the patient to Dr Patel (Cardiology SpR)

Situation – My name is Dr_____ and I am the FY2 in A&E. I have just seen Mr Rhodes, a 75 year old gentleman who presents with a third degree heart block and haemodynamic instability.

Background – Mr Rhodes has a history of ischaemic heart disease. He has come into A&E complaining of severe difficulty in breathing, fatigue, dizziness and feeling generally unwell.

Assessment – His initial observations were HR: 30 Regular. BP: 90/60. RR: 32 SaO_2: 90 % (RA) Temp 36.9 °C. He was pale, clammy and had peripheral cyanosis. CRT was 4 seconds. His heart rate was 30. ECG showed a characteristic trace of 3rd degree complete heart block.

I have given him high flow oxygen, obtained IV access and given him a fluid challenge. He has received intravenous atropine. His heart rate and blood pressure have improved following treatment to HR 46, BP 100/70.

Recommendation – I would like you to review this patient with regards to his complete heart block.

Bradycardia in brief:

1. What is bradycardia?
Bradycardia is defined as an adult heart rate of less than 60 beats per minute. It has many causes, including athletic fitness, certain medications, sinus node dysfunction in the elderly, hypothyroidism, hypothermia, hypoxia, pericardial tamponade or atrioventricular block.

2. What is the management of bradycardia?
The management of bradycardia depends on the cause and severity. If the patient is severely symptomatic, haemodynamically compromised or has a heart rate of less than 40 they will need treatment with a muscarinic antagonist atropine or beta-agonists such as isoprenaline (should only be given with senior supervision). If the patient fails to respond to initial medical therapy temporary transcutaneous pacing may be required. Certain patients will benefit from a permanent pacemaker.

3. What are the types of atrioventricular (AV) blocks?
There are 4 main types of AV blocks:
- First-degree - constant prolonged PR interval.
- Second-degree Mobitz type 1 - increasing length of the PR interval until a QRS complex does not follow a P wave.
- Second-degree Mobitz type 2 - periodically missed QRS complexes despite regular P waves (2:1; 3:1).
- Third-degree complete heart block - P waves and QRS complexes occur independently of each other.

Case 8 – **Cardiac Tamponade**

You are a Foundation Year 2 doctor working in the Emergency Department. Mr Rocco, a 57 year old gentleman, comes in complaining of shortness of breath, anxiety, fatigue, and a fast heart beat. He is currently not in any pain. He has a known history of lung cancer, but is unable to give you any further information.

Please conduct an A to E assessment of Mr Rocco and commence the initial management.

Latest observations:
HR: 128. BP: 84/64. RR: 34 SaO_2: 85 % (RA) Temp 36.9 °C UO: NA

Danger

It is safe to approach Mr Rocco

Response

Mr Rocco is alert and responsive

Airway

Look – Nothing is seen obstructing the airway
Feel – Trachea is not deviated
Listen – Normal breath sounds
Treat – The patient is maintaining his airway, no treatment is necessary

Breathing

Look – Severely dyspnoeic, pale, clammy
Feel – Chest expansion and percussion normal
Listen – Bilateral inspiratory crackles in the lower lung zones.
Measure – RR 34, SaO_2 85 % (RA)
Treat – High flow oxygen should be offered. Call for senior help at this stage
Reassess – Patient is still dyspnoeic but SaO_2 is now 95 %

Further investigations:
- ABG - type 1 respiratory failure
- Chest X-ray - large cardiac silhouette with pulmonary oedema

Circulation

Look – Pale, clammy, peripheral cyanosis, large distended neck veins with a raised JVP of 8 cm.
Feel – Cool peripheries, apex beat not displaced, CRT 4 seconds
Listen – Muffled heart sounds, pericardial friction rub heard
Measure - HR: 128. BP: 84/64. Temp 36.9 °C
Treat – obtain IV access, give a fluid challenge. Call for senior assistance as this patient will require a pericardiocentesis. Following a discussion with your seniors consider giving ionotropes such as dobutamine. This patient will have to be managed in high dependency settings
Reassess – HR 125. BP 94/67. Temp 36.9 °C. Patient appears to be improving

Further investigations:
- ECG - sinus tachycardia, small voltage QRS complexes, electrical alternans
- Echocardiogram - large pericardial effusion (if available in the Emergency Department)
- Bloods (FBC, U&E, LFT, CRP, Troponin, BNP, CK)

Prominent distended neck veins with a raised JVP, hypotension and muffled heart sounds are known as Beck's Triad. Though a rare constellation of signs, this suggests a diagnosis of acute cardiac tamponade. The management of cardiac tamponade involves obtaining intravenous access, giving fluids and inotropic drugs such as dobutamine, and definitive management involves performing a pericardiocentesis under ultrasound guidance.

Disability

AVPU – Patient alert and fully responsive/GCS 15
Blood glucose – 5.7 mmol/L
Pupils – Equal and reactive to light

Exposure

Fully expose the patient and perform a detailed head to toe examination. Hepatomegaly is found on abdominal examination.

Hand over the patient to Dr Patel (Cardiology SpR)

Situation – My name is Dr_____ and I am the FY2 in A&E. I have just seen Mr Rocco, a 57 year old gentleman with a cardiac tamponade leading to cardiogenic shock.

Background - Mr Rocco presented with shortness of breath, anxiety, fatigue, and fast palpitations. He has a known history of lung cancer.

Assessment – His observations were HR: 128. BP: 84/64. RR: 34 SaO_2: 85 % (RA) Temp 36.9 °C. On examination, he was severely dyspnoeic, pale and clammy. He had peripheral cyanosis, large distended neck veins with a raised JVP of 8 cm as well as muffled heart sounds with a pericardial friction rub. He had hepatomegaly on abdominal examination. A chest x-ray showed an enlarged cardiac silhouette with pulmonary oedema, and an echo showed a large pericardial effusion. I suspected cardiac tamponade and obtained IV access, gave him high flow oxygen, and fluids. Following this his observations have slightly improved.

Recommendation – I would like you to review this patient, and consider giving him dobutamine and performing an ultrasound-guided pericardiocentesis as definitive management, and investigate the cause of his cardiac tamponade. Is there anything else you would like me to do in the meantime?

Cardiac tamponade in brief:

1. What is a cardiac tamponade?
Cardiac tamponade occurs when there is an accumulation of fluid, blood or gas in the pericardial space. The heart is then unable to expand and fill as per normal, resulting in a decreased cardiac output. Hence the patient often experiences anxiety, fatigue, dyspnoea, tachypnoea and tachycardia. The reduced cardiac output also leads to a decrease in perfusion of the peripheries and may cause cardiogenic shock.

2. What is the management of a cardiac tamponade?
Cardiac tamponade is a medical emergency and needs to be treated quickly. The immediate management involves giving fluids and inotropic drugs such as dobutamine. The definitive management involves performing a pericardiocentesis under ultrasound guidance. Recurrent pericardial effusions and tamponade can be managed surgically.

3. What are the common causes of a cardiac tamponade?
The underlying cause should always be investigated. Common causes of a cardiac tamponade include malignancies (e.g. lung cancer), trauma, infections especially HIV, TB and viral pericarditis, connective tissue diseases (SLE), acute and chronic kidney disease (uraemic pericarditis), radiation and myxoedema of hypothyroidism.

Gastrointestinal and Surgical Emergencies

Janice Lee

Acute Upper Gastrointestinal Bleeding	84
Acute Pancreatitis	88
Spontaneous Bacterial Peritonitis and Sepsis	94
Ulcerative Colitis and Toxic Megacolon	100
Splenic Rupture	104
Ruptured Abdominal Aortic Aneurysm	110
Strangulated Hernia	114

Case 1 – **Acute Upper Gastrointestinal Bleeding**

You are the Foundation Year 2 doctor working in the Emergency Department. A 65 year old gentleman, Mr Kent, has been brought in by ambulance. The patient is unable to give a history but the ambulance crew tell you that they were called by his wife as he had three episodes of vomiting fresh bright red blood this morning.

Please conduct an A to E assessment of Mr Kent and commence the initial management.

Latest observations:
HR: 120 BP: 90/55 RR: 20 SaO_2: 96 % (room air) Temp: 37.5 °C UO: NA

Danger

It is safe to approach the patient. Be aware of spillages and bodily fluids, such as blood on the floor, and wear an apron and gloves.

Response

The patient is responsive but appears confused.

Airway

The airway is patent as the patient is calling out for his wife

Breathing

Look – breathing rapidly but no use of accessory muscles
Feel – trachea is central, chest expansion is symmetrical, percussion is resonant
Listen – vesicular breath sounds throughout, no added sounds
Measure – RR: 20 SaO_2: 96 % (RA)
Treat – Move on

Circulation

Look – pale, no active haematemesis, dry mucous membranes
Feel – cool and clammy, regular rapid pulse with reduced volume
Listen – normal heart sounds
Measure – HR: 120 BP: 90/55 CRT 3s UO: NA
Treat – Insert two large-bore cannulae, fluid resuscitate with intravenous crystalloid (up to 30ml/kg); insert a urinary catheter (for fluid balance monitoring)
Reassess – HR: 100 BP: 100/60 CRT 2 secs UO: 30 mL/hr

Further investigations:
- ECG monitoring (sinus tachycardia)
- ABG - metabolic acidosis with a raised lactate and a haemoglobin of 80 g/L
- Bloods (FBC, U&E, LFT, glucose, clotting screen, amylase/lipase)
- Crossmatch 4 – 6 units of packed red blood cells. Consider activating major haemorrhage protocol

Disability

AVPU – Alert/GCS 14 (E4, V4, M6)
Blood glucose – 4 mmol/L
Pupils – Equal and reactive to light

Exposure

Fully expose the patient and look for signs of chronic liver disease (eg. telangiectasia, purpura, jaundice), perform abdominal and digital rectal examination which identifies melaena. The patient does not have any evidence of chronic liver disease. Keep the patient nil by mouth.

Consider performing an erect chest radiograph to exclude an oesophageal or bowel perforation.

Calculate the patient's Blatchford score (see below).

Hand over to Dr Gill (Gastroenterology registrar)

Situation – Hello Dr Gill, my name is _____ and I am the FY2 in A&E. I am calling about a 65 year old gentleman with an acute upper GI bleed.

Background – His name is Mr Kent and he was brought into A&E by ambulance having had three episodes of haematemesis this morning. He was conscious but confused so I was not able to get a history or any medical background.

Assessment – On examination he was pale and his peripheries were cold and clammy. He was tachycardic at 120/min and his BP was 90/55, which has responded to a 500mL fluid challenge. His HR is now 100/min and BP has come up to 100/60. On examination, he did not have any signs of chronic liver disease but there was melaena on the digital rectal examination. His Blatchford score is___. He has two large-bore cannulae with resuscitation fluids running. I have taken bloods including a crossmatch, ordered a chest x-ray to exclude a perforation and catheterised him.

Recommendation – I would like you to come and review this patient. I suspect he needs an urgent endoscopy and I have kept him nil by mouth. I do not have any evidence to suspect that this might be a variceal bleed so I would like your advice on terlipressin and antibiotics. Is there anything else you would like me to do?

Acute upper gastrointestinal bleed in brief

1. What are the common causes of an acute upper gastrointestinal bleed?
- Peptic ulcer disease
- Oesophagitis/gastritis/duodenitis
- Oesophago-gastric varices
- Mallory-Weiss tear

2. What are the Blatchford and Rockall scoring systems?
These are scoring systems recommended for all patients with an acute upper GI bleed to enable early risk stratification. Blatchford score at first assessment and the full Rockall score after endoscopy. There are multiple online calculators which allow you to accurately calculate both.

The Blatchford bleeding score is based on clinical and laboratory variables. A score of 0 identifies low-risk patients who may be suitable for outpatient management. The variables used include:
- Blood urea
- Haemoglobin
- Systolic blood pressure
- Pulse rate
- Presentation with melaena or syncope
- Hepatic disease
- Cardiac failure

The full Rockall score uses clinical criteria (age, shock, co-morbidities) and endoscopic findings to help predict the risk of re-bleeding and mortality. Patients with a full score of <3 have a low risk of re-bleeding or death and should be considered for early discharge and outpatient follow-up.

3. What is the management of an acute variceal bleed?
1. Get help from your seniors.
2. Resuscitate until haemodynamically stable (consider red cell transfusion after loss of ≥30 % of circulating volume or Hb<10 in ongoing bleeds).
3. Correct clotting abnormalities with vitamin K, fresh frozen plasma and a platelet transfusion.
4. Start terlipressin infusion prior to endoscopy, and continue it after endoscopic treatment.
5. Start prophylactic antibiotic therapy (according to your hospital guidelines)
6. Arrange endoscopy immediately after resuscitation so that an appropriate intervention can be done (banding or sclerotherapy).
7. High-dose intravenous proton pump inhibitor therapy should be used following successful endoscopic haemostatic therapy.
8. If bleeding is uncontrolled, a Sengstaken-Blakemore tube should be considered as a temporary salvage treatment. Transjugular intrahepatic portosystemic stent shunting is recommended as the long-term solution.

Case 2 – **Acute Pancreatitis**

You are a Foundation Year 2 doctor working in the Emergency Department. A 56 year old woman, Mrs Hill, has been brought in by ambulance complaining of severe epigastric pain that radiates to the back, nausea and vomiting. She has a history of alcohol excess.

Please conduct an A to E assessment of Mrs Hill and commence the initial management.

Latest observations:

HR: 110 BP: 100/70 RR: 16 SaO_2: 100 % (room air) Temp: 37.8 °C UO: NA

Danger
It is safe to approach the patient.

Response
The patient is responsive but is distressed and in a lot of pain.

Airway
It is safe to assume airway is patent.

Breathing
Look – no signs of respiratory distress
Feel – trachea is central, chest expansion is symmetrical, and percussion is resonant
Listen – decreased breath sounds in both bases
Measure – RR: 16 SaO_2: 100 % (room air)
Treat – move on

Circulation
Look – JVP not raised, no pallor, moist mucous membrane
Feel – sweaty, regular rapid pulse, normal skin turgor
Listen – normal heart sounds
Measure – HR: 110 BP: 100/70 Temp: 37.8 °C CRT 2 secs UO: NA
Treat – Insert two large-bore cannulae, IV crystalloid infusion (to counter third-space sequestration), keep nil by mouth, insert a urinary catheter (to monitor fluid balance)
Reassess – HR: 100 BP: 110/80 Temp: 37.3 °C CRT 2 s UO: 60 mL/hr

Further investigations:
- ECG (sinus tachycardia)
- Arterial blood gas
- Erect chest x-ray and abdominal x-ray (to exclude perforation or obstruction)
- Abdominal ultrasound scan (to look for gallstones)
- Bloods (FBC, U&E, LFT, calcium, clotting screen, amylase/lipase, lipid profile)

Disability
AVPU – Alert/GCS 15 (E4, V4, M6)
Blood glucose – 4.5 mmol/L
Pupils – Equal and reactive to light

Exposure

Fully expose the patient and perform an abdominal examination. The patient is very tender in the epigastrium. Also look for bruising over the umbilical area and the flanks. There is jaundice and scleral icterus. Prescribe analgesia.

Further investigations:
- Request an abdominal ultrasound and consider an abdominal CT scan

Calculate Glasgow score (see below).

Hand over to Mr Patel (Surgical registrar)

Situation – Hello Mr Patel, my name is _____ and I am the FY2 in A&E. I am calling about a 56 year old lady who presented with an acute abdomen and I'm worried it may be acute pancreatitis. She has a significant alcohol abuse history.

Background – Her name is Mrs Hill and she presented with a two-day history of severe epigastric pain that radiated to her back, associated with nausea and vomiting.

Assessment – On initial assessment, she was tachycardic at 105 with a BP of 100/70. She was sweaty and jaundiced and tender in the epigastrium. I have inserted two large-bore cannulae, taken blood and done an ABG which was normal. Her Glasgow score is___. I have started IV fluids and analgesia, kept her nil by mouth and requested an erect chest x-ray and an abdominal ultrasound.

Recommendation – Could you please come and assess this patient and advise on whether she needs a nasogastric tube and prophylactic antibiotics? Is there anything else you would like me to do in the meantime?

Acute pancreatitis in brief

1. What scoring system is frequently used for acute pancreatitis?

Modified Glasgow criteria for predicting severity of pancreatitis (validated for pancreatitis caused by gallstones and alcohol).

	CRITERIA	POSITIVE VALUE
P	PaO$_2$	<8 kPa
A	Age	>55 years
N	Neutrophils	WCC >15x10^9/L
C	Calcium	<2 mmol/L
R	Renal function	Urea >16 mmol/L
E	Enzymes LDH AST	>600 iu/L >200 iu/L
A	Albumin (serum)	<32 g/L
S	Sugar (blood glucose)	>10 mmol/L

Three or more positive factors within 48 hours of onset suggest severe pancreatitis and high risk of complications. These patients should be managed in intensive care settings. Other predictors of a severe attack are obesity (BMI >30), pleural effusion on a chest radiograph and CRP >150 mg/L.

Other scoring systems are Ranson's criteria, which has been validated for alcohol-induced pancreatitis and can only be fully applied after 48 hours, the Acute Physiology and Chronic Health Examination (APACHE)-II criteria, and the Bedside Index for Severity in Acute Pancreatitis (BISAP) criteria.

2. What are the common causes of acute pancreatitis?
- Gallstones (50 %)
- Alcohol (20 %)
- Idiopathic (20 %)
- Drugs (5 %) e.g. steroids, furosemide, azathioprine
- Viral infection e.g. mumps, HIV
- Hypertriglyceridaemia, hypothermia, hypercalcaemia
- Endoscopic retrograde cholangiopancreatography (ERCP)

3. What are the complications of acute pancreatitis?
Local complications:
- Inflammatory mass
- Infected necrosis
- Pancreatic pseudocyst formation
- Pseudo-aneurysm
- Obstructive jaundice
- Gastric outflow obstruction
- Portal vein thrombosis
- Chronic pancreatitis

Systemic complications
- Sepsis
- Pleural effusion
- Acute respiratory distress syndrome
- Acute renal failure
- Disseminated intravascular coagulopathy

Case 3 – **Spontaneous Bacterial Peritonitis and Sepsis**

You are a Foundation Year 1 doctor working on the gastroenterology ward. The ward nurse asks you to urgently review Mr White who is complaining of severe abdominal pain. Mr White, a 45-year-old gentleman was admitted three days ago with jaundice, anorexia, malaise and severe ascites. He is known to have decompensated alcoholic liver disease.

Please conduct an A to E assessment of Mr White and commence the initial management.

Latest observations:
HR: 120 BP: 90/55 RR: 21 SaO$_2$: 96 % (room air) Temp: 38.5 °C UO: NA

Danger
It is safe to approach the patient.

Response
The patient is responsive.

Airway
It is safe to assume the airway is patent.

Breathing
Look – Breathing rapidly but no use of accessory muscles
Feel – Trachea is central, chest expansion is symmetrical, percussion is resonant
Listen – Vesicular breath sounds throughout, no added sounds
Measure – RR: 21 SaO$_2$: 96 % (room air)
Treat – Consider giving oxygen if sepsis is suspected and patient is critically unwell

Circulation
Look – Sweaty, not cyanosed, JVP not raised, moist mucous membranes
Feel – Cool peripheries, regular rapid pulse
Listen – Normal heart sounds
Measure – HR: 120 BP: 90/55 Temp: 38.5 °C CRT 2 secs UO: NA
Treat – Insert two large-bore cannulae, initial fluid challenge with a crystalloid solution (in patients with chronic liver disease fluids should be used cautiously and senior advice should be obtained). insert a urinary catheter to monitor output; paracetamol for pyrexia.
Reassess – HR: 100 BP: 110/70 Temp: 38.5°C CRT: 2 s UO: 50 mL/hr

Further investigations:
- ECG (sinus tachycardia)
- Bloods (FBC, U&E, LFT, CRP, glucose, clotting, amylase/lipase, ammonia)
- Blood cultures
- Urine dip stick and send off sample for microbiology
- Perform a venous blood gas (metabolic acidosis with a raised lactate)

Disability
AVPU – Alert/GCS 15
Blood glucose – 6 mmol/L
Pupils – Equal and reactive to light

Exposure

Fully expose the patient and look for possible sources of infection (do not forget to check for intravascular lines or skin rashes, and take samples for microbiology if needed).

Perform an abdominal examination – you note signs of decompensated chronic liver disease (eg. oedema, telangiectasia, purpura, jaundice), a distended abdomen with guarding, rigidity and rebound tenderness. Shifting dullness is elicited. On digital rectal examination there is no melaena or masses.

The patient appears septic. Give intravenous empirical antibiotics after taking blood cultures (e.g. tazocin and gentamicin, but do refer to your local guidelines) and continue paracetamol (see Box 1).
Consider a CT abdomen pelvis to check for intra-abdominal pathology.

Hand over to Dr Roberts (Gastroenterology registrar)

Situation – Hello Dr Roberts, my name is _____ and I am the FY1 on the gastroenterology ward. I am calling about a patient on the ward who has become septic and possibly has spontaneous bacterial peritonitis.

Background – His name is Mr White, a 45 year old gentleman who was admitted to the ward three days ago with malaise, anorexia, jaundice and severe ascites. He has a background of decompensated alcoholic liver disease. An hour ago he started to feel unwell and complained of severe abdominal pain.

Assessment – On examination he had a temperature of 38.5 and HR 120 with a BP of 90/55. He had ascites with guarding, rigidity and rebound tenderness. A venous blood gas showed a metabolic acidosis with a raised lactate. I have taken bloods including culture, catheterised him and started him on resuscitation fluids and IV antibiotics as per hospital guidelines. I am also considering a CT abdomen pelvis.

Recommendation – I would like you to come and review this patient urgently. I suspect he needs an ascitic tap to confirm the diagnosis and guide further antibiotic therapy. Is there anything else you would like me to do?

> **Box 1. The "Sepsis Six"**
>
> The 'Sepsis Six' includes doing the following within one hour if sepsis is suspected:
> 1. Give high-flow oxygen
> 2. Take blood cultures
> 3. Give intravenous antibiotics according to local protocol
> 4. Start intravenous fluid resuscitation with a crystalloid (e.g. NaCl 0.9% or Hartmann's solution)
> 5. Check lactate
> 6. Monitor hourly urine output and consider catheterisation

Spontaneous bacterial peritonitis and sepsis in brief

1. How do you define sepsis and septic shock?

Sepsis

Sepsis occurs when a dysregulated host response to a pathogen causes severe organ dysfunction. Organ dysfunction in this case can be defined using the Sequential Organ Failure Assessment (SOFA) score, requiring 2 or more of
- A systolic blood pressure of less than or equal to 100 mmHg
- An altered mental state with a GCS of less than 15
- A respiratory rate of more than or equal to 22

Septic shock

For a patient to be diagnosed with septic shock the following two criteria are required:
- Persistent hypotension despite fluid resuscitation and vasopressor use
- A lactate of 2 mmol/L or more

Patients with septic shock have a very high in hospital mortality (>40%).

2. What is the management for ascites in chronic liver disease?
1. Fluid restriction (<1.5 L/day)
2. No added salt to food and low salt diet (40 – 100 mmol/day)
3. Spironolactone to counter the deranged renin-angiotensin-aldosterone axis (+/- furosemide if there is poor response, closely monitor renal function)
4. Therapeutic paracentesis with concomitant 20 % human albumin infusion
5. Transjugular intrahepatic portosystemic shunt (TIPSS)
6. Liver transplantation is the definitive treatment

3. What is spontaneous bacterial peritonitis (SBP)?
SBP is an acute bacterial infection of ascitic fluid that affects approximately 10 % of patients with cirrhotic ascites. Bacterial translocation, bacteraemia, and impaired antimicrobial activity of ascitic fluid contribute to its development. It should be suspected in any patient with ascites who deteriorates clinically, even in the absence of abdominal pain and pyrexia. A diagnosis of SBP is confirmed by a white cell count >250/mm^3 in aspirated ascitic fluid. It is treated with intravenous antibiotics.

Case 4 – **Ulcerative Colitis and Toxic Megacolon**

You are the Foundation Year 1 doctor working on the gastroenterology firm. Mr Thomas, a 28 year old with a background of ulcerative colitis, was admitted with a 3-day history of bloody diarrhoea, fever and vomiting. A nurse has asked you to urgently review the patient, as he has developed severe abdominal pain and has become drowsy.

Please conduct an A to E assessment of Mr Thomas and commence the initial management.

Latest observations:
HR: 125 BP: 90/55 RR: 25 SaO_2: 99 % (room air) Temp: 38.5 °C UO: NA

Danger
It is safe to approach the patient.

Response
The patient is responsive but appears drowsy

Airway
He is complaining of severe abdominal pain. It is safe to assume the airway is patent.

Breathing
Look – the patient has rapid breathing but no use of accessory muscles
Feel – trachea is central, chest expansion is symmetrical, percussion is resonant
Listen – vesicular breath sounds throughout, no added sounds
Measure – RR: 25, SaO$_2$: 100 % (RA)
Treat – Move on

Further investigations:
- Perform a VBG (metabolic acidosis with a raised lactate)
- Order an erect chest x-ray (air under the diaphragm)

Circulation
Look – pale, distressed, dry mucous membranes
Feel – sweaty, regular rapid pulse, reduced volume, reduced skin turgor
Listen – normal heart sounds
Measure – HR: 125 BP: 90/55 Temp: 38.5 °C, CRT: 3 secs UO: NA
Treat – Insert two large-bore cannulae, fluid challenge with 500ml 0.9 % NaCl, up to 2000 ml, insert urinary catheter (for careful fluid balance)
Reassess – HR: 110 BP: 105/82 Temp: 38.5 °C CRT: 2 secs UO: 30 mL/hr

Further investigation:
- Bloods (FBC, U&E, LFT, CRP, calcium, glucose, clotting screen, amylase/lipase)
- Blood cultures
- Group & Save 2 – 4 units of packed red blood cells
- Consider a CT abdomen pelvis

Disability

AVPU – Alert/GCS 14 (E4, V4, M6)
Blood glucose – 5.5 mmol/L
Pupils – Equal and reactive to light

Exposure

Fully expose the patient and look for possible sources of infection. Perform an abdominal examination: patient's abdomen is slightly distended with no signs of chronic liver disease. It is tender throughout with rebound tenderness and rigidity. Bowel sounds are absent.

Order a CT abdomen pelvis (following a discussion with your senior), which shows a toxic megacolon and free air in the abdomen suggestive of a perforation. Keep patient nil by mouth. The patient appears septic, therefore give intravenous antibiotics after taking blood cultures (e.g. tazocin and gentamicin, but do follow your local guidelines) and paracetamol.

Hand over to Mr Bailey (Surgical SpR)

Situation – Hello Mr Bailey, my name is _____ and I am the FY1 on the gastro-enterology ward. I am calling about a 28 year old gentleman with known ulcerative colitis whom I'm worried may have toxic megacolon with a perforation.

Background – His name is Mr Thomas and he was admitted with a 3-day history of bloody diarrhoea, fever and vomiting.

Assessment – He was tachycardic, pyrexic with a low blood pressure. On examination, his abdomen was distended and tender throughout, with rebound tenderness and rigidity. Bowel sounds were absent and the digital rectal exam showed fresh blood. A venous blood gas showed a metabolic acidosis with a raised lactate. I have taken bloods including cultures, group and saved 4 units of packed red blood cells and commenced resuscitation fluids. Both an erect chest x-ray and a CT abdomen pelvis demonstrated free air in the abdomen consistent with a perforation.

Recommendation – I would like you to come and assess this patient urgently as I think he may need a laparotomy. Is there anything else you would like me to do in the meantime?

Ulcerative colitis and toxic megacolon in brief

1. What criteria can be used to assess severity of ulcerative colitis (UC)?
The Truelove & Witts criteria assist in determining the severity of ulcerative colitis flare up. Please refer to the table below.

VARIABLE	MILD	MODERATE	SEVERE
Motions/day	<4	4 – 6	>6
Rectal bleeding	Small	Moderate	Large
T°C at 6 am	Apyrexial	37.1 – 37.8	>37.8
Resting pulse (bpm)	<70	70 – 90	>90
Haemoglobin (g/L)	>110	105 – 110	<105
ESR (mm/h)	<30		>30

2. What is toxic megacolon?
Toxic megacolon refers to acute toxic colitis with dilatation (total or segmental) of the colon. It is defined radiologically as a transverse colonic diameter of >6cm with loss of haustration. It occurs in about 5 % of cases of severe UC and can be triggered by opiates or hypokalaemia.

3. What are some causes of toxic megacolon?
- Inflammatory (ulcerative colitis, Crohn's colitis, pseudomembranous colitis)
- Infectious (eg. Salmonella, Shigella, Campylobacter, Clostridium difficile, Entamoeba histolytica, cytomegalovirus)
- Radiation colitis
- Ischaemic colitis
- Nonspecific colitis secondary to chemotherapy

4. How is toxic megacolon managed?
The aim of treatment is to (1) reduce colonic distension to prevent perforation; (2) correct fluid and electrolyte disturbances and (3) treat toxaemia and precipitating factors.

During initial resuscitation, give fluid and electrolyte replacement and transfuse as necessary. Initiate broad-spectrum IV antibiotics and IV steroids. Stop all medications that may affect colonic motility (e.g. antidiarrhoeals, anticholinergics, opiates), place the patient on bowel rest and insert a nasogastric tube to assist with decompression. Closely monitor the patient and repeat abdominal x-ray every 12 hours.

Indications for urgent colectomy are free perforation, massive haemorrhage, increasing toxicity and progression of colonic dilatation. Patients who do not improve after 24 – 72 hours of maximal medical therapy should have colectomy because of the high risk of perforation.

Case 5 – **Splenic Rupture**

You are a Foundation Year 2 doctor working in the Emergency Department. Mr Fred Brown, a 36 year old gentleman is brought in by ambulance complaining of severe left upper abdominal pain. He had flu-like symptoms and a sore throat for the past 2 weeks and his GP made the diagnosis of infectious mononucleosis due to EBV. An hour ago Fred collapsed after his usual judo training session.

Please conduct an A to E assessment of Mr Brown and commence the initial management.

Latest observations:

HR: 130 BP: 80/40 RR: 22 SaO_2: 98 % (room air) Temp: 36.7 °C UO: NA

Danger
It is safe to approach the patient.

Response
The patient is responsive but appears drowsy. You should call for senior help at this stage.

Airway
The patient is talking; therefore it is safe to assume airway is patent.

Breathing
Look – The patient is tachypnoeic and using accessory muscles of respiration
Feel – Trachea is central, chest expansion is symmetrical, percussion is resonant
Listen – Vesicular breath sounds throughout, no added sounds
Measure – RR: 22 SaO$_2$: 98 % (room air)
Treat – High flow oxygen and move on

Circulation
Look – Pale, JVP not visible
Feel – Cold peripheries, regular rapid reduced volume pulse
Listen – Normal heart sounds
Measure – HR: 130 BP: 80/40 Temp: 36.7 °C; CRT: 5 secs UO: NA
Treat – Insert two large-bore cannulae, resuscitate with crystalloid (fluid challenge with 500 ml up to 2000 ml), insert a urinary catheter
Reassess – HR: 110 BP: 100/60 Temp: 36.8 °C CRT: 2 secs UO: 20 mL/hr

Further investigations:
- ECG (sinus tachycardia)
- Bloods (FBC, U&E, LFT, clotting screen, amylase)
- Activate your hospital's Major Haemorrhage Protocol and take blood samples from cross-match

Disability

AVPU – Alert/ GCS 14 (E4, V4, M5)
Blood glucose – 5.1 mmol/L
Pupils – Equal and reactive to light

Exposure

Fully expose the patient and examine from head to toe. Perform an abdominal examination – abdomen rigid and tender in the left upper quadrant with localised peritonism (rigidity and guarding), and splenomegaly. ENT examination – erythematous tonsils but no pus, enlarged cervical lymph nodes.

Further investigations:
- FAST scan: Homogenous splenomegaly with subcapsular haematoma and intraperitoneal fluid
- Contrast CT scan demonstrates perisplenic fluid collection, with the spleen displaced by mass effect consistent with splenic rupture. (See Box 1)

Hand over to Mr Anderson (Surgical SpR)

Situation – Hello Mr Anderson, my name is _____ and I am the FY2 in A&E. I am calling about a 36 year old gentleman, Mr Brown, who has a splenic rupture.

Background – He presented with left upper quadrant pain radiating to the left shoulder after collapsing at a judo training session. For the past 2 weeks he has had fever, sore throat, dry cough and flu-like symptoms, and the GP made the diagnosis of infectious mononucleosis.

Assessment – The patient was tachycardic at 130 bpm, hypotensive with a BP of 80/40 and peripherally shut down. His abdomen was rigid and tender, particularly in the left upper quadrant. An abdominal ultrasound showed splenomegaly, subcapsular haematoma and intraperitoneal fluid. I have commenced him on resuscitation fluids, taken bloods including a crossmatch and activated the hospital's major haemorrhage protocol.

Recommendation – Could you please come and assess this patient urgently as I think he has ruptured his spleen and may need to go to theatre. Is there anything else you would like me to do in the meantime?

> **Box 1. Management options of splenic rupture**
> - Non-operative (active observation)
> - Angioembolisation using mechanical (metal coils, embolisation particles) or chemical (Gelfoam, sclerosant chemicals, thrombin) agents
> - Splenectomy

Splenic rupture in brief

1. What are the indications for a splenectomy?
- Splenic trauma
- Spontaneous rupture (e.g. splenomegaly caused by EBV infection)
- Hypersplenism
- Autoimmune haemolysis (e.g. immune thrombocytopenic purpura or warm autoimmune haemolytic anaemia)
- Congenital haemolytic anaemia

2. What are some post-splenectomy complications?
- Temporary increase in circulating white blood cells and platelets predisposing to thrombi
- Diminished responsiveness to some vaccines
- Increased susceptibility to infection by bacteria (especially encapsulated bacteria eg. Haemophilus influenzae type b, Neisseria meningitidis and Streptococcus pneumoniae) and protozoa

3. What advice and precautions must be given to post-splenectomy patients?
- Immunisations:
- Pneumococcal vaccine: two weeks pre-op or two weeks after emergency splenectomy. Re-immunise every 5 years. Avoid in pregnancy.
-Haemophilus influenzae type b vaccine
-Meningococcal A,B,C,W,Y vaccines
- Annual influenza vaccine
- Lifelong prophylactic oral antibiotics (phenoxymethypenicillin or erythromycin if penicillin allergic) to high risk groups (<16 or >50 years, inadequate serological response to pneumococcal vaccination, history of previous invasive pneumococcal disease, splenectomy performed for haematological malignancy)
- Emergency supply of antibiotics
- Medical alert card, pendants or bracelets to alert medical staff
- Advice to seek medical attention if any signs of infection

Case 6 – **Ruptured Abdominal Aortic Aneurysm**

You are a Foundation Year 2 doctor working in the Emergency Department. Mr Rossi, a 65 year old gentleman is brought in by the paramedics, unconscious. The paramedics say Mr Rossi complained of sudden-onset severe abdominal pain radiating to his back before fainting. Mr Rossi has been awaiting an elective repair of his abdominal aortic aneurysm.

Please conduct an A to E assessment of Mr Rossi and commence the initial management.

Latest observations:
HR: 145 BP: 80/55 RR: 29 SaO$_2$: 92 % (room air) Temp: 37.0 °C UO: NA

Danger

It is safe to approach the patient.

Response

The patient is unresponsive. Call for help and put out an arrest call.

Airway

Look – No signs of airway obstruction (e.g. foreign body, vomitus, oedema)
Feel – Movement of air felt against cheek
Listen – No stridor, snoring, gurgling, choking or coughing
Treat – Perform a head tilt and chin lift, consider inserting an oropharyngeal airway
Reassess – Airway secure

Breathing

Look – The patient is tachypnoeic with central cyanosis
Feel – Trachea is central, chest expansion is symmetrical, percussion is resonant
Listen – Vesicular breath sounds throughout, no added sounds
Measure – RR: 29 SaO$_2$: 92 % (room air)
Treat – High-flow oxygen (15L/min) via non-rebreathe mask
Reassess - RR: 22 SaO$_2$: 100 %

Further investigations:
- Perform an ABG – raised anion gap metabolic acidosis, lactate 7 and a haemoglobin of 80g/L

Circulation

Look – Conjunctival pallor, cyanosed, dry mucous membranes
Feel – Cool and clammy, regular rapid pulse, reduced volume, reduced skin turgor, weak peripheral pulses in the legs
Listen – Normal heart sounds
Measure – HR: 145 BP: 80/55 Temp: 37.0 °C CRT: 4 secs UO: NA
Treat – Insert two large-bore cannulae, give 250-500 mL boluses of fluid challenges, insert a urinary catheter
Reassess – HR: 120 BP: 90/60 Temp: 37.0 °C CRT: 5 seconds UO: 25 mL/hr

The patient responds poorly to the fluid challenge. You should seek help from your seniors immediately.

Further investigations:
- ECG – sinus tachycardia
- Bloods (FBC, U&E, LFT, clotting screen)
- Activate your hospital's Major Haemorrhage Protocol and cross-match blood

Disability

AVPU – Unresponsive/GCS 7 (E1, V2, M4)
Blood glucose – 6.0 mmol/L
Pupils – Equal and reactive to light

The patient's GCS is 7 and he therefore needs intubation for a definitive airway. You should be getting in touch with the anaesthetic team immediately.

Exposure

On abdominal examination – pulsatile and expansile abdominal mass felt. Abdominal ultrasound scan may show free fluid. CT should only be done if the patient is stable.

> Haemodynamically unstable patients with a suspected ruptured abdominal aortic aneurysm should be taken to theatre without delay.

Hand over to Mr Marsh (Vascular surgery SpR)

Situation – Hello Mr Marsh, my name is ___ and I am the FY2 in A&E. I am calling about a 65 year old gentleman with suspected ruptured abdominal aortic aneurysm.

Background – His name is Mr Rossi and he was brought in unconscious and shocked. He is known to have an abdominal aortic aneurysm and complained of sudden-onset severe abdominal and back pain before collapsing.

Assessment – He was unresponsive and tachypnoeic with a RR of 29 and SaO_2 of 92 %. ABG showed a raised anion gap metabolic acidosis with a raised lactate. He is cold and clammy with weak peripheral pulses. His HR: 145 BP: 80/55 and cap refill: 5 secsonds. I have activated the hospital's major haemorrhage protocol and commenced him on resuscitation fluids. Since his GCS was 7, the anaesthetists have intubated him. An abdominal USS showed free fluid.

Recommendation – I think this patient needs immediate intervention. Can you come and see him urgently? In the meantime I will ring the theatre staff. Is there anything else you would like me to do?

> **Box 1. Management of Abdominal Aortic Aneurysm (AAA)**
>
> Ruptured AAA requires immediate surgical intervention. Untreated, mortality is 100 %. Elective repair is recommended for aneurysms ≥5.5cm, or those expanding at >1cm/year or symptomatic aneurysms.
>
> Types of repair for AAA:
> - Surgical (open) repair: Involves exposure of the abdominal aorta, aortic and iliac clamping and replacement of the aneurysmal segment with a prosthetic graft.
> - Endovascular aneurysm repair (EVAR): Involves introducing a stent-graft system through the femoral arteries, which relines the aneurysm, diverts blood flow through the endograft and allows the aneurysm to thrombose.

Abdominal aortic aneurysm (AAA) in brief

1. What is an aortic aneurysm?
An aneurysm is a permanent and irreversible dilatation of a blood vessel by at least 50 % of the normal expected diameter. Aortic aneurysms are classified as abdominal or thoracic.

An abdominal aortic aneurysm (AAA) is defined as aortic diameter >3 cm. Most AAAs arise below the level of the renal arteries, but can involve the renal ostia and arise supra-renally.

2. What are the common risk factors for abdominal aortic aneurysms?
- Male sex
- Increasing age
- Family history
- Peripheral atherosclerotic vascular disease
- Hypertension
- Hyperlipidaemia
- Smoking
- Increased weight

3. What screening programmes are advised for abdominal aortic aneurysms?
The AAA Screening Programme invites men for screening during the year that they turn 65. Screening involves an ultrasound scan of the abdomen that usually takes less than 10 minutes.

Frequency of AAA screening:
- Diameter of 3 - 3.9cm - screen every 3 years
- Diameter of 4 - 4.4cm - screen every 2 years
- Diameter of 4.5 - 5.4cm - screen every year

Case 7 – **Strangulated Hernia**

You are a Foundation Year 2 doctor working in the Emergency Department. Mr Thompson, a 56 year old gentleman, presents with a six hour history of a severely painful lump in his right groin. He is known to have a right inguinal hernia and is awaiting elective repair.

Please conduct an A to E assessment of Mr Thompson and commence the initial management.

Latest observations:
HR: 110 BP: 130/80 RR: 16 SaO$_2$: 96 % (room air) Temp: 37.0 °C UO: NA

Danger
It is safe to approach the patient.

Response
The patient is responsive and appears to be in severe pain.

Airway
It is safe to assume airway is patent.

Breathing
Look – No evidence of respiratory distress
Feel – Trachea is central, chest expansion is symmetrical, percussion is resonant
Listen – Vesicular breath sounds throughout, no added sounds
Measure – RR: 16 SaO_2: 94 % (room air)
Treat – Move on

Circulation
Look – No pallor, moist mucous membrane
Feel – Sweaty, regular rapid pulse, normal skin turgor
Listen – Normal heart sounds
Measure – HR: 110 BP: 130/80 Temp: 37.0 °C Cap refill: 2 secs UO: NA
Treat – Insert a cannula, commence IV fluids and offer pain relief (i.e. morphine)

Further investigations:
- VBG - metabolic acidosis with a raised lactate suggesting bowel ischaemia
- Bloods (FBC, U&E, LFT, CRP, coagulation) including Group & Save

Disability
AVPU – Alert/GCS 15
Blood glucose – 5.3 mmol/L
Pupils – Equal and reactive to light

Exposure
Fully expose the patient and examine from head to toe. Perform an abdominal examination – mildly distended abdomen, diffusely tender. There is a non-reducible tender, erythematous swelling in the right groin with no cough impulse, no lumps on the left side. 'Tinkling' bowel sounds.

Further investigations:
- Abdominal x-ray – multiple loops of distended small bowel seen centrally
- CT abdomen - to check the anatomy and level of obstruction as well as the viability of the remaining bowel

Insert an NG tube and keep nil by mouth.

Hand over to Mr Morgan (Surgical registrar)

Situation – Hello Mr Morgan, my name is _____ and I am the FY2 in A&E. I am calling regarding a 56 year old gentleman with a suspected strangulated right inguinal hernia with small bowel obstruction.

Background – His name is Mr Thompson and he came in with a six-hour history of severe pain in his right groin and one episode of vomiting. He is known to have a right inguinal hernia and was awaiting elective repair.

Assessment – His initial observations were within normal limits. On examination his abdomen was mildly distended and diffusely tender. There was a non-reducible and very tender erythematous swelling in the right groin. There were no lumps on the left side. An abdominal X-ray showed multiple loops of distended small bowel centrally. I have taken bloods, inserted an NG tube and started IV fluids. I have also made him nil by mouth.

Recommendation – I would like you to come and review this patient as he may require immediate surgical intervention. Is there anything else you would like me to do?

Hernias in brief

1. What is a hernia?
It is the protrusion of a viscus or part of a viscus through a defect in the walls of its containing cavity into an abnormal position. The defect may be congenital or acquired.

There are some risk factors that predispose an individual to acquiring a hernia such as chronic cough, chronic constipation, obesity, surgery and severe muscular effort (e.g. heavy lifting)

2. What are the different terms used to describe abdominal hernias?
- Reducible – its content can return to the abdominal cavity either spontaneously or with manipulation.
- Irreducible – the hernia cannot be reduced despite pressure or manipulation.
- Incarcerated – the hernia is irreducible due to adhesions within the sac, without obstruction or strangulation.
- Obstructed – the bowel within the hernia is obstructed.
- Strangulated – the blood supply to the hernia contents is occluded by pressure at the neck of the hernia. This can lead to impaired viability of the bowel if the bowel is within the sac.

3. What is the anatomy of the inguinal canal?
- **Superiorly** - internal oblique and transverse abdominis muscle
- **Anteriorly** - external oblique aponeurosis and internal oblique
- **Inferiorly** - inguinal and lacunar ligaments
- **Posteriorly** - transversalis fascia

4. What are the contents of the inguinal canal?
- **Females** - round ligament of the uterus and the ilioinguinal nerve
- **Males** - spermatic cord (made up of three fascial layers: external spermatic, cremasteric, and internal spermatic)

  Contents of the spermatic cord:
- Three arteries: artery to vas deferens, testicular artery, cremasteric artery
- Pampiniform venous plexus
- Vas deferens
- Lymphatics
- Genital branch of the genitofemoral nerve
- Autonomic nerves

5. What are the two types of inguinal hernia?

INDIRECT INGUINAL HERNIA	DIRECT INGUINAL HERNIA
The most common form (80 % of inguinal hernias, especially in children).	More common in the elderly, rare in children.
Passes through the deep inguinal ring along the inguinal canal.	Protrudes directly through a weakness in the posterior wall of the inguinal canal.
Runs lateral to the inferior epigastric vessels.	Runs medially to the inferior epigastric vessels.

Neurological Emergencies

Zhi Min Yap

Meningitis	122
Stroke	128
Status Epilepticus	136
Subarachnoid Haemorrhage (SAH)	142
Extradural Haemorrhage (Head Injury)	146

Case 1 – **Meningitis**

You are a Foundation Year 1 doctor working on the acute medical ward. Mr. Smith is a 79-year-old man admitted acutely unwell from a nursing home with a high temperature, a throbbing headache that started yesterday and two episodes of vomiting. His carers have not observed any changes in his mood or behaviour, but report that he has been low in energy for the past 3 weeks.

Please conduct an A to E assessment of Mr. Smith and commence the initial management.

Latest observations:
HR: 110 BP: 110/80 RR: 20 SaO_2: 98 % (RA) Temp: 39.0 °C UO: NA

Danger
It is safe to approach the patient.

Response
The patient appears very confused but is responsive to voice.

Airway
Mr. Smith tells you he is nauseous and has a bad headache. The pain travels down his neck and is worse when he looks at the light. It is safe to assume the airway is patent.

Breathing
Look – Rapid breathing
Feel – Trachea is central, equal chest expansion, resonant to percussion bilaterally
Listen – Vesicular breathing throughout, no added sounds
Measure – RR: 20, SaO_2: 98 % (RA)
Treat – The patient's SaO_2 is satisfactory at this point so there is no need for supplementary oxygen. Start continuous pulse oximetry monitoring and consider giving oxygen if his saturations drop below <94 %.

Circulation
Look – Sweaty, not cyanosed, JVP not elevated, dry mucous membranes
Feel – Cool extremities, regular rapid pulse with normal volume, reduced skin turgor
Listen – Normal heart sounds
Measure – HR: 110, BP: 110/80 Temp: 39.0 °C Cap refill: 3 secs UO: NA
Treat – Obtain IV access, give anti-pyretics, maintenance fluids and IV antibiotics
Reassess – Temp: 38.5 °C

Further investigations:
- Bloods (FBC, U&E, LFT, CRP, glucose, clotting screen, lactate)
- Blood cultures before antibiotics within the first hour of presentation
- Send urine sample for microbiology
- ECG (sinus tachycardia)
- Lumbar puncture once raised intracranial pressure is ruled out with a CT head scan.

Disability
AVPU – patient is responsive to voice/GCS 13 (E3V4M6)
Capillary blood glucose – 6 mmol/L
Pupils – equal and reactive to light, patient is extremely photophobic

Exposure

Fully expose the patient and perform a detailed secondary examination.
No rash is noted and his abdomen is soft and non-tender.

On examination, there is nuchal rigidity and passive knee extension with the hips flexed causes pain and resistance (Kernig's sign). No papilloedema on fundoscopy.

This patient demonstrates red flag signs of meningeal irritation and is septic and therefore requires immediate treatment with antibiotics which should not be delayed (see Box 1). He is at risk of deteriorating and hence a senior review should be sought urgently.

Hand over the patient to Dr Patel (Medical SpR)

Situation – This is Dr____, the F1 on the Acute Medical Unit. I have just reviewed Mr. Smith, a 79 year old gentleman who presents with headache, fever and photophobia. He is septic and I suspect he has meningitis.

Background – Mr Smith was previously well and was admitted from a nursing home. His carers report he has been increasingly tired over the past three weeks and became acutely unwell overnight. There are no concerns about acute behavioural changes.

Assessment - On examination, he is only responsive to voice and appears unwell. He is photophobic with a stiff neck and a positive Kernig's sign. His pupils are reactive and there is no papilloedema. I have secured intravenous access, sent off bloods and cultures as part of his septic work up and commenced maintenance fluids and empirical antibiotics. His blood pressure is stable. I have also placed a request for an urgent CT scan prior to a lumbar puncture, but because of his low GCS he will need to be accompanied by an anaesthetist.

Recommendation – I suspect Mr. Smith has meningitis. He is very unwell and I am worried he will deteriorate. I would like you to review him urgently with a view of performing a lumbar puncture following his CT head scan. Is there anything else you would like me to do?

> **Box 1. Management of Meningitis**
>
> Request for a CT head scan prior to performing a lumbar puncture to exclude mass effect, which could lead to coning if CSF pressure is released during a tap. Initiate empirical antibiotic therapy for meningitis: ceftriaxone, (add ampicillin for patients >55 years old). If penicillin-allergic use chloramphenicol. However, do consult your local hospital guidelines. Perform a lumbar puncture and send the CSF for microscopy, culture and sensitivity, glucose (with a simultaneous paired serum sample), cytology, cell count and PCR.

Meningitis in brief

1. What is meningitis? How is it different from meningococcal disease?

Meningitis refers to the inflammation of the meninges. This is distinct from encephalitis, which is inflammation of the brain parenchyma itself. Inflammation can involve both structures where it is then known as meningoencephalitis. The extent of inflammation can be hard to define at initial presentation – clinical features that point towards encephalitis include an insidious onset, changes in behaviour, altered consciousness levels, and when focal neurology or seizures are preceded by an infectious prodrome. When encephalitis is suspected, consider treating empirically with antivirals (e.g. acyclovir) before the exact cause is known, as mortality in untreated viral encephalitis is high ≈70 %.

Meningococcal disease refers specifically to the disease caused by Neisseria meningitidis, a Gram-negative diplococcus usually found as a bacterial commensal in the nasopharynx. This is the leading cause of infectious death in children under the age of five and is a notifiable disease in the UK. Meningococcal disease can present with meningitis (15 %), septicaemia (25 %) or a combination of both (60 %).

2. What causes meningitis and what are some risk factors?

The causes of meningitis can be broadly classified into infectious and non-infectious. Infectious causes predominate, and are most commonly viral in nature, but can also be bacterial, fungal or protozoal. Each class of pathogens gives rise to characteristic CSF findings (Table 1.) and more specific tests like PCR can also be performed to identify the underlying agent. The specific pathogens causing meningitis vary according to age, hence empirical antibiotic therapy differs between neonates, adults and the elderly.

	Appearance	White cells/µL	Protein mg/dL	Glucose
Normal	Clear	0-5	<0.45	>60 % of serum level
Bacterial meningitis	Cloudy, turbid	> 100 (neutrophils)	>50	<40% of serum level
Viral Meningitis	Clear	10 - 1000 (neutrophils early on, then lymphocytes)	>50	>60% (may be low in herpes infection)
Tuberculous meningitis	Clear	50 – 500 (neutrophils early on, then lymphocytes)	>50 (may be normal)	<40% of serum level
Fungal Meningitis	Clear or cloudy	10-500	>50	<40% of serum level

In a traumatic tap, allow 1 white blood cell for every 500 red blood cells, and 0.1g/L of protein for every 1000 red cells.
Normal white cell counts do not rule out meningitis.
Always interpret CSF glucose with a paired serum glucose sample taken simultaneously.

Table 1. Characteristic cerebrospinal fluid (CSF) findings in adult meningitis. Note that these values may vary at the extremes of age. Other tests to consider : Gram stain, Zeihl Neelsen and auramine stains, India ink stain, direct bacterial antigen detection, and PCR for specific viral pathogens.

3. What is the management of meningitis?

The mainstay of treatment is urgent antimicrobial therapy to minimise long-term complications like deafness and neurocognitive sequelae. Dexamethasone may also be given in children with bacterial meningitis, but should not be given in cases of septic shock or known meningiococcal disease.

Empirical antibiotics should be commenced before the specific organisms causing the infection are known. These include cephalosporins (cefotaxime or ceftriaxone) with the potential addition of amoxicillin or ampicillin. In penicillin allergic patients, chloramphenicol may be used.

Case 2 – **Stroke**

You are a Foundation Year 2 doctor working in the Emergency Department. Mr Walker is a 75-year-old gentleman brought in with acute onset right arm weakness. He was out for a jog 30 minutes ago when he suddenly developed right arm weakness and collapsed. He is currently not in any pain and does not report any headache or photophobia. He denies any previous episodes of weakness. His past medical history is notable for hypertension, hypercholesterolaemia and atrial fibrillation. He takes ramipril 10 mg BD, simvastatin 40mg nocte and has never taken anticoagulants. He has no known drug allergies.

Please conduct an A to E assessment of Mr. Walker and commence the initial management.

Latest observations:

HR: 93 BP: 155/90 SaO$_2$: 98 % (room air) Temp: 36.9 °C UO: NA

Danger

It is safe to approach Mr Walker.

Response

Mr. Walker is alert and responsive. His right arm is lying completely still, although he is moving his left arm normally.

Airway

Mr. Walker has expressive dysphasia – it is safe to assume his airway is patent.

His speech is spontaneous but he has difficulty in finding words. If you have a high clinical suspicion of a stroke at this point, keep the patient nil by mouth until a complete neurological and swallow assessment is performed to avoid any potential aspiration.

Breathing

Look – Tar stains noted on his fingers. No signs of respiratory distress
Feel – Trachea is central with symmetrical chest expansion
Listen – Chest is clear on auscultation
Measure – RR 18 SaO$_2$ 98 % (RA)
Treat – His breathing is stable. Start continuous pulse oximetry and consider O$_2$ supplementation if SaO$_2$ drops to <94 % . It is important to avoid hypoxia in patients with suspected stroke

Circulation

Look – JVP is not elevated, no peripheral oedema
Feel – Warm peripheries, pulse is irregularly irregular in rate and volume
Listen – Normal heart sounds. No carotid bruits audible (this does not rule out a carotid source of emboli)
Measure – HR 93 BP 155/90 CRT 2 secs Temp 36.9 UO – not available.
Treat – Obtain intravenous access and commence maintenance fluid (avoid overhydration due to the risk of cerebral oedema). Maintain normothermia – use oral or IV paracetamol and blankets as needed.

Further Investigations:
- Perform an ECG
- Bloods (FBC, U&E, LFT, lipids, coagulation)

His blood pressure should not be reduced in the acute setting unless an aortic dissection is suspected or there are signs of hypertensive encephalopathy. A drop in BP may compromise cerebral perfusion as autoregulation is already impaired. It is noteworthy that a BP of >220/130 is a contraindication to thrombolysis, and the BP should be maintained below 185/110 for 24 hours after thrombolysis.

Disability

AVPU – Patient is alert / GCS 15 (E4V5M6)
Capillary Blood glucose – 6 mmol/L
Pupils – Equal and reactive to light, there is no papilloedema on fundoscopy.

Hypoglycaemia must always be excluded as the cause for sudden onset neurological symptoms. Ensure tight blood sugar control between 4 – 11 mmol/L. Use insulin infusion if diabetic or if blood sugars are not well-controlled. Both hyperglycaemia and hypoglycaemia can mimic an ischaemic stroke, as well as aggravate ongoing neuronal damage.

Exposure

There are no signs of bleeding or bruising elsewhere. The patient does not have a stiff neck or photophobia. On examination of his neurological system:
- General inspection – there is no facial asymmetry and his speech is fluent and spontaneous but slurred.
- Gait – normal.
- Tone – reduced in right arm, normal in left arm and lower limbs.
- Power – MRC 0/5 in right arm, 5/5 in left arm and lower limbs.
- Reflexes – diminished in the right arm only.
- Coordination – unable to assess right arm, intact elsewhere. No cerebellar signs noted (nystagmus, intention tremor, staccato speech).
- Sensation – fine touch and proprioception are grossly intact.
- Cranial Nerves – right homonymous hemianopia, conjugate gaze is intact.

He has a ROSIER score of 4, making the diagnosis of an acute stroke likely – the stroke team must be contacted IMMEDIATELY (see Box 1) and the patient should have an urgent CT head scan.

Box 1. **Diagnosis and Management of Stroke**

ROSIER SCALE
*if BM <3.5 mmol/L treat urgently and reassess once blood glucose is normal

	YES (+/-1)	NO (0)
Has there been loss of consciousness or syncope?	-1	0
Has there been seizure activity?	-1	0
Is there NEW ACUTE ONSET (or on awakening from sleep)?		
i. asymmetric facial weakness	+1	0
ii. asymmetric arm weakness	+1	0
iii. asymmetric leg weakness	+1	0
iv. speech disturbance	+1	0
v. visual field defect	+1	0

*Stroke is likely if total scores are >0. Scores of </= 0 have a low possibility of stroke but it is not completely excluded.

Mr. Walker is having an acute stroke affecting his right arm which started 30 minutes ago. As he is between 8 – 80 years old and is seen within 4.5 hours of the onset of his symptoms, he is a potential candidate for thrombolysis with IV recombinant tissue plasminogen activator (tPa: e.g. alteplase). The next priority would be to get an urgent CT head scan to rule out a primary haemorrhage, and work him up for urgent thrombolysis within 4.5 hours of symptom onset. If the CT scan is normal but there is a high clinical suspicion of a stroke, consider a diffusion-weighted MRI, which is better at visualising posterior fossa lesions (brainstem/cerebellum).

Thrombolysis should be administered in a stroke unit with immediate access to re-imaging facilities, where staff are trained in the delivery of thrombolysis and management of potential complications. Appropriately trained emergency medicine staff may also administer alteplase provided patients can subsequently be managed within a stroke service. Every patient treated with alteplase must have a repeat CT head scan after 24 hours of thrombolysis, and given aspirin 300 mg after 24 hours for 14 days, unless contraindicated.

Hand over the patient to Dr. Patterson (Stroke SpR)

Situation – Hi, I am Dr._____ , the FY2 in the A&E department. I have just reviewed Mr. Walker, a 75-year-old male who presented with a 30 minute history of isolated right arm weakness and expressive dysphasia following a collapse. I think he is having a left-sided stroke and may be a candidate for thrombolysis.

Background – His past medical history is significant for several vascular risk factors including hypertension, hypercholesterolaemia and atrial fibrillation. He had no strokes or TIAs in the past. He is not on any anticoagulation at the moment.

Assessment – His current observations are RR: 18 HR: 93 BP: 155/90 SaO$_2$: 98 % (RA) Temp: 36.9 °C. I have assessed him and he is cardiovascularly stable at the moment. Assessing his neurological status, he has isolated reduced tone, power (MRC 0/5) and reflexes in his right arm with intact sensation. His cranial nerves are normal apart from a right-sided homonymous hemianopia. These findings are consistent with a left sided infarct.

I have started continuous cardiac monitoring and requested for hourly neurological observations with blood glucose monitoring. His blood glucose is now 6mmol/L and he is not known to have diabetes. I have started him on maintenance fluid and will be monitoring his hydration status closely. I have requested for an urgent CT head scan to rule out a primary haemorrhagic stroke.

Recommendation – Mr. Walker is a having a stroke that started 30 minutes ago. I would be grateful if you could assess him urgently as a potential candidate for thrombolysis and for transfer to the hyperacute stroke unit.

Stroke in brief

1. What is the definition of a stroke?

A stroke is defined as acute onset of focal neurological deficit, resulting from the disruption of cerebral blood flow due to ischaemic infarction or bleeding into a part of the brain. This is in contrast to a transient ischaemic attack (TIA) where the focal neurological symptoms last <24 hours (often much shorter) due to temporary occlusion of a part of the cerebral circulation. Because a TIA cannot be confidently diagnosed unless the symptoms have resolved within 24 hours, those who present with ongoing neurological symptoms and signs suggestive of an acute stroke or TIA should be treated as if they have a stroke.

The ROSIER scale is used for stroke assessment only. Patients with no intial abnormal neurology should be evaluated with the ABCD2 score (see Table 1.) to identify those at high risk of developing a stroke after a TIA. The objective is to prevent recurrence or a complete stroke.

		POINTS
A – age	>60 years old	1
B – blood pressure	BP at presentation >140/90 mmHg	1
C – clinical features	Unilateral weakness	2
	Speech disturbance without weakness	1
D – duration of symptoms	>60 minutes	2
	10 – 59 minutes	1
D – diabetes	Diabetic	1
		Total: 0 – 7

- Criteria for specialist assessment and investigation within 24 hours: ABCD2 >/=4 or crescendo TIA (>2 TIA in a week) regardless of ABCD2 score.
- Cases with ABCD2 <4 should be reviewed in a specialist TIA clinic within 1 week of presentation. If the history is compatible with a TIA, start aspirin 300 mg OD immediately.

Table 1. ABCD2 prognostic score for suspected TIA.

2. What are the contraindications for thrombolysis?

The window of opportunity for effective thrombolysis is 4.5 hours from the onset of symptoms. As 20% of strokes are haemorrhagic, this must be excluded with urgent neuroimaging prior to thrombolysis. Other contraindications to thrombolysis include (the list is not exhaustive):
- Recent surgery or trauma
- Previous central nervous system haemorrhage
- Seizures at presentation
- Platelet count <100 x 10^9/L
- Current anticoagulation (INR >1.7)
- Severe hypertension
- Known intracranial malignancy
- Known bleeding disorder or active bleeding on presentation

3. How can strokes be classified according to the clinical presentation?

The presenting features of a stroke can point towards the area of infarction in the brain, and this can be a significant prognostic factor. Broadly, strokes can be classified into four cerebral infarction syndromes under the Bamford classification (see Table 2.). Total anterior circulation infarcts (TACI) have the worst prognosis in terms of mortality and morbidity, while posterior circulation infarcts, partial anterior circulation infarcts (PACI) and lacunar infarcts have better prognoses on the whole.

CEREBRAL INFARCTION SYNDROMES	VESSELS AFFECTED	CLINICAL FEATURES
Total Anterior Circulation Infarct (TACI)	Total occlusion of middle cerebral artery AND anterior cerebral artery	All THREE of: 1. Unilateral weakness (and/or sensory deficit) of face, arm and leg 2. Homonymous hemianopia 3. Higher cerebral dysfunction e.g. dysphasia/ dysarthria
Partial Anterior Circulation Infarct (PACI)	Branch occlusions of middle cerebral artery and/or anterior cerebral artery	TWO of: 1. Unilateral weakness (and/or sensory deficit) of face, arm and leg 2. Homonymous hemianopia Higher cerebral dysfunction e.g. dysphasia
Posterior Circulation Infarct	Posterior cerebral artery	ONE of: 1. Cerebellar or brainstem syndrome* 2. Loss of consciousness 3. Isolated homonymous hemianopia.
Lacunar Syndrome (LACS)	Subcortical infarct due to occlusion of small penetrating vessels, often due to hypertension	There is no evidence of higher cerebral dysfunction. This can be further subclassified into: 1. Pure motor stroke 2. Pure sensory stroke 3. Pure sensorimotor stroke 4. Ataxic hemiparesis (combined cerebellar and pyramidal signs in the same limb)

* Depending on the areas affected (i.e. the cranial nerve nuclei, the cranial nerves and/or the long tracts within the brainstem) brainstem strokes can present in a variety of ways. There are a number of eponymous syndromes associated with damage to particular areas of the brainstem, e.g. lateral medullary syndrome (Wallenberg's) comprises contralateral loss of pain and temperature sensation in the trunk and limbs (crossing of spinothalamic tracts), with ipsilateral loss of these sensory modalities in the face.

Table 2. The Bamford Stroke Classification

Case 3 – **Status Epilepticus**

You are a junior doctor in the Emergency Department. A 25-year-old female is brought in by ambulance. She collapsed and started seizing in the shopping center 30 minutes ago. On arrival, she is still seizing with generalized tonic-clonic jerking movements in all 4 limbs. Her medical history is unknown and your colleague is getting more information from the witnesses at the moment.

Please conduct an A to E assessment of this patient and commence the initial management.

Latest observations:

HR 110 BP: 120/80, SaO_2: 90 % (room air), Temp: 37.0 °C, UO: NA

Danger

It is safe to approach the patient. Sharp objects in the vicinity have been removed.

Response

The patient is unconscious and actively seizing in all four limbs. She does not appear malnourished or unkempt and does not smell of alcohol.

Airway

Look – The patient is unconscious and not able to protect her airway. There are no foreign bodies or vomit obstructing her airway. She does not have dentures or other dental appliances.
Feel – The patient's breath can be felt against your cheek.
Listen – There are no abnormal breath sounds (gagging/gurgling/ stridor/ snoring) audible.
Treat – Open the airway by laying the patient in a semiprone recovery position. Consider a nasopharyngeal airway or intubation if the airway becomes compromised. It is unlikely that you will be able to insert an oropharyngeal airway in someone who is actively seizing, as they would have clenched their jaws.
Reassess – Frequently reassess airway for signs of obstruction

Breathing

Look – Patient is breathing rapidly. There is no peripheral or central cyanosis.
Feel – Symmetrical chest expansion, trachea is central.
Listen – Chest is clear on auscultation – there is no evidence of an aspiration
Measure – RR: 20 SaO$_2$ 90 % (RA)
Treat –Administer 15 L oxygen via a non-rebreathe mask with target saturations of 94 – 98 %.
Reassess – RR 20, O$_2$ Sats 100 % on 15 L O$_2$

Further investigations
• Arterial blood gas – type 1 respiratory failure with a raised lactate

The ABG can aid in identifying potential reversible causes of seizures like electrolyte abnormalities (low Na$^+$), acute hypoxia, and drug overdoses, which may present with a raised anion gap metabolic acidosis. The ABG is also vital to monitor for worsening of lactic acidosis. However, a raised lactate is normal in patients who are seizing.

Circulation

Look – Pale, no cyanosis.
Feel – Warm and sweaty.
Listen – Normal heart sounds.
Measure – HR 110, BP: 120/80 CRT : 2 seconds, Temp: 37.0 °C UO: NA
Treat – Obtain IV access. Administer antiepileptic medication (buccal midazolam or IV lorazepam).
Reassess – the patient stops seizing (re-examine the patient from the beginning)

Further Investigations:
- Perform an ECG (sinus tachycardia)
- Bloods (FBC, U&Es, LFT, CRP, glucose, calcium, magnesium, coagulation)
- Blood anticonvulsant levels
- Full toxicology screen

Request for continuous cardiac monitoring (BP, ECG) and pulse oximetry particularly as anti-epileptic treatment has been given. Phenytoin can cause a drop in BP and is contraindicated in bradycardia or heart block. Close monitoring of respiratory function is required with benzodiazepines, particularly in patients who have never taken benzodiazepines before.

Disability

AVPU – Patient is unresponsive/ GCS 5 (E1V1M3)
Capillary blood glucose – 6 mmol/L
Pupils – equal and reactive to light. There is no papilloedema on fundoscopy.

The patient has a GCS of 5 and may require intubation. An anaesthetist should therefore be informed and the patient's airway closely monitored. She will have to be managed on a critical care unit.

Exposure

Examining the patient from head to toe, there are no signs of head trauma, meningism or focal neurological deficit. Consider an urgent CT scan if head injury is suspected to be a precipitant.

Ensure there is no evidence of secondary trauma resulting from the seizure.

There are no medic alert bracelets/ necklaces visible.

The diagnosis of a tonic-clonic status epilepticus is usually clear. After basic life support, the next priority is to terminate the seizures as soon as possible to minimize the risk of brain damage and death (see Box 1).

Box 1. Management of Status Epilepticus

Commonly used anti-epileptic agents include
i. Benzodiazepines (require close respiratory monitoring)
    a. Buccal midazolam
    b. Intravenous lorazepam - can be repeated until seizures stop or 20 mg given in total. Give second dose if no response within 2 minutes
ii. Phenytoin infusion – if seizures persist despite benzodiazepines. Will require continuous ECG and BP monitoring. Check phenytoin levels to guide loading and maintenance doses.

If seizures remain refractory to the above treatment, the patient will require admission to ITU, intubation and induction with a general anaesthetic (e.g. propofol, thiopental) with continuous EEG monitoring.

When performing the A to E assessment, one should focus on identifying reversible causes of seizures like hypoglycaemia, alcohol intoxication and electrolyte abnormalities. Thiamine can be given if alcoholism or malnourishment is suspected. Treat hypoglycaemia with intravenous glucose. As glucose increases the risk of Wernicke's encephalopathy, thiamine should always be given beforehand in patients with suspected alcohol excess.

Hand over the patient to Dr Mohammed (Critical Care SpR)

Situation – Hello, I am Dr._____ , the FY2 in the A&E department. I have just seen a 25-year-old female who was brought in with status epilepticus.

Background – Her identity and past medical history are unknown at the moment.

Assessment – Her airway was at risk and she was desaturating on room air. I therefore inserted a nasopharyngeal airway and gave her high flow oxygen, which improved her saturations to 98%. Her seizures were terminated with intravenous lorazepam. She is haemodynamically stable but her current GCS is 5. She is being reviewed by the anaesthetist for consideration of intubation. We have sent off blood anticonvulsant levels and toxicology screen. Her blood glucose is 6 and her pupils are equal and reactive to light.

Recommendation – Would you be able to review this lady? Is there anything else you would like me to do in the meantime?

Status epilepticus in brief:

1. What is status epilepticus?
Status epilepticus is defined as seizures lasting for more than 30 minutes, or repeated episodes of seizures that occur without the patient regaining consciousness in between. It is a medical emergency with high rates of mortality and risks of permanent brain damage with increasing duration of seizures.

2. What are the potential medical complications of status epilepticus?
With increasing duration of seizures, the patient is at risk of developing secondary complications such as:
- Hypoxia
- Lactic acidosis
- Hypoglycaemia
- Arrhythmias (complication of treatment with phenytoin)
- Rhabdomyolysis
- Electrolyte abnormalities (particularly Na^+/K^+)
- Hyper- or hypotension
- Raised intracranial pressure

Patients with status epilepticus require close cardiac and respiratory monitoring, to ensure prompt treatment of these complications as they arise.

Case 4 – **Subarachnoid Haemorrhage (SAH)**

You are a junior doctor in the Emergency Department. Mr. Thompson, a 35 year old lawyer, is brought in by ambulance with a severe throbbing headache that came on suddenly as though he had been hit on the back of his head. The headache came on without any warning 30 minutes ago while he was at work and peaked in intensity within seconds of onset. On arrival he is mildly confused, nauseous, dizzy and bent over with his head in his hands. He is complaining of photophobia and neck stiffness. His medical history is unremarkable and he does not suffer from regular headaches. There is no history of recent trauma.

Please perform an A to E assessment of this patient and commence the initial management.

Latest observations:
HR 120 BP: 130/90, SaO$_2$: 96 % (RA), Temp: 36.9 °C, UO: NA

Danger

It is safe to approach the patient.

Response

The patient is responsive to voice. He appears mildly confused.

Airway

Mr. Thompson answers your questions in full sentences and tells you he would like some pain relief as the headache is unbearable. It is safe to assume his airway is patent.

Breathing

Look – Patient is breathing rapidly. There is no peripheral or central cyanosis
Feel – Symmetrical chest expansion, trachea is central
Listen – Chest is clear on auscultation
Measure – RR: 20 SaO$_2$: 98 % (RA)
Treat – No treatment is required at this point. Start continuous pulse oximetry monitoring and give oxygen if saturations drop to <94 %, with target SaO$_2$ of 94 – 98 %

Circulation

Look – Pale
Feel – Warm and sweaty, peripheral pulses are intact – regular and tachycardic
Listen – Normal heart sounds
Measure – HR 120, BP: 130/90 CRT : 2 seconds, Temp: 37.0°C UO: NA
Treat – Secure intravenous access. Offer appropriate pain relief (e.g. paracetamol and codeine phosphate). Prescribe anti-emetics as required (e.g. metoclopramide or domperidone). Do not give antisteroidals to someone with suspected subarachnoid haemorrhage

Further investigations:
- Continuous cardiac monitoring (blood pressure, ECG)
- Bloods (FBC, LFT, U&E, clotting)

Disability

AVPU – Patient is responsive to voice with a GCS of 13/15 (E3V4M6)
Capillary blood glucose – 6 mmol/L
Pupils – equal and reactive to light. Patient is photophobic. There is no papilloedema on fundoscopy – this is often a late sign of raised intracranial pressures.

Exposure

There is no evidence of bleeding or trauma elsewhere. On examination of his neurological system, Mr. Thompson has a stiff neck with no other focal neurological deficits. In particular, he has full range of eye movements and does not have a third nerve palsy, which may raise concerns of a posterior communicating artery aneurysm or raised intracranial pressure and brainstem herniation.

> A subarachnoid haemorrhage is a neurological emergency. Initiate regular neurological observations to detect any deterioration which may occur secondary to cerebral ischaemia, rebleeding or acute hydrocephalus.

The priority after stabilising the patient during an A to E assessment is to confirm the diagnosis. Request an urgent CT head scan – this will confirm the diagnosis in 95 % of patients within 24 hours of presentation. The sensitivity of CT imaging decreases beyond this time window, and a lumbar puncture looking for xanthochromia (as evidence of blood in the CSF) may be required if the CT is normal but the history is highly suggestive of SAH.

As soon as the diagnosis is confirmed, Mr. Thompson should be discussed with the neurosurgical unit regarding the necessary treatment (neurosurgery or endovascular intervention). Oral nimodipine should be given to reduce cerebral vasospasm and prevent rebleeding and cerebral ischaemia.

Hand over to Mr. Smith (Neurosurgical SpR)

Situation – Hi Mr. Smith, my name is _____ and I am the FY2 in A&E. I would like to refer Mr. Thompson, a 35 year old gentleman who has a subarachnoid haemorrhage, which was confirmed on a CT scan.

Background – Mr. Thompson is normally fit and well with no medical history of note. He does not have regular headaches and denies any recent trauma. He is not on any regular medications and has no known allergies. He was brought in by ambulance with a sudden onset severe headache associated with nausea, photophobia and neck stiffness that started 30 minutes ago while he was at work.

Assessment – His current observations are HR 120 BP: 130/90, SaO$_2$: 96 % (RA), Temp: 36.9 °C. He has a GCS of 13/15 (E3V4M6). He has neck stiffness but no focal neurological deficit. I have initiated regular neurological observations to monitor for any deterioration. I have prescribed pain relief and anti-emetics as required, secured intravenous access and sent bloods off for FBC, LFT, U&E and clotting. A CT head confirmed SAH and he was started on oral nimodipine.

Recommendations – Mr. Thompson has a subarachnoid bleed and I would like you to review him urgently to determine whether any neurosurgical input is required. Is there anything else you would like me to do in the meantime?

Subarachnoid haemorrhage (SAH) in brief

1. What are some red flag features that distinguish SAH from other headaches?
A thunderclap headache (that is the first and worst ever in someone without a past history of headaches) suggests a subarachnoid bleed. Some patients may experience 'herald bleeds' during which they report distinct severe headaches in the preceding days/weeks before the main SAH bleed. These patients are often misdiagnosed as having migraines, so a high degree of clinical suspicion is required. Cluster headaches are often very severe (10/10 intensity) and can mimic a SAH. The nature of the pain is unilateral and peri-orbital, often waking the patient up from sleep at night.

2. What are the causes of a SAH?
Common causes include a ruptured aneurysm (70 %), arterio-venous (AV) malformations (5 %) and no cause is identified in up to 20 %. Other rare causes include space-occupying lesions, vasculitis, and trauma with associated cerebral contusion.

3. What are the prognostic features of a SAH?
The severity of SAH can be assessed by the symptoms at presentation with the Hunt and Hess Scale (Grade 1 – 5). Patients should be frequently reassessed to detect any neurological deterioration, which carries a worse prognosis.

GRADE	SYMPTOMS	SURVIVAL
1	Asymptomatic, mild headache	70 %
2	Moderate to severe headache, neck stiffness, no neurological deficit except cranial nerve palsy	60 %
3	Drowsy	50 %
4	Stuporous, hemiparesis	20 %
5	Coma, decerebrate rigidity	10 %

Table 1. The Hunt and Hess Scale

Case 5 – **Extradural Haemorrhage (Head Injury)**

You are a Foundation Year 2 doctor working in the Emergency Department. Mr Nowak is a 33 year old construction worker who is brought in by ambulance after he blacked out after taking a hit on the head at work an hour ago, whilst not wearing a helmet. He regained consciousness 2 minutes later but is now very lethargic. He has a persistent headache and is feeling nauseous. He has a vague memory of being hit but has no recollection of the events leading up to his admission. Mr Nowak is normally fit and well. The paramedics have immobilised his cervical spine. Your colleague is taking a history from his co-workers regarding the circumstances around the injury.

Please perform an A to E assessment of this patient and commence the initial management.

Latest observations:

HR: 100 BP: 130/90, RR: 21 SaO_2: 96 % (room air) Temp: 36.9 °C UO: NA

Danger

It is safe to approach the patient.

Response

The patient is responsive to voice but appears drowsy.

Airway

It is safe to assume the airway is patent.

Breathing

Look – He does not appear to be in respiratory distress
Feel – Trachea is central. Chest expansion is equal and symmetrical. Percussion is resonant bilaterally
Listen – Chest is clear to auscultation.
Measure – RR 18, SaO$_2$ 96 % (room air)
Treat – He does not require oxygen at this point. Initiate continuous pulse oximetry

Circulation

Look – Well perfused
Feel – Peripheries are warm to touch
Listen – Normal heart sounds
Measure – HR 100 BP 130/80 Temp: 36.9°C UO: NA
Treat – Prescribe pain relief and anti-emetics as required

Further investigation:
- Bloods (FBC, LFT, U&E, clotting, Group & Save)

Disability

AVPU – Patient is responsive to voice with a GCS of 13/15 (E3V4M6)
Capillary blood glucose – 6 mmol/L
Pupils – equal and reactive to light. There is papilloedema on fundoscopy.

You should raise this patient's head of the bed. If the patient deteriorates or shows signs of tentorial herniation, inform on-call neurosurgeons urgently. Intracranial pressure can be further reduced by intravenous mannitol and hyperventilation – this requires intubation and paralysis, hence the patient should be discussed with ITU early on.

Exposure

Expose the patient fully. Look for bruises behind the ear (Battle's sign), bleeding from the ears (otorrhoea) or CSF rhinorrhoea (if present these would suggest a base of skull fracture). The presence of a skull fracture greatly increases the likelihood of an intracranial haematoma.

On examination of his neurological system, his cranial nerves are intact with a normal resting eye position and a full range of spontaneous eye movements. He has reduced power in his left arm and leg (MRC 3/5) with intact sensation throughout.

Further investigations:
- CT head (right extradural haematoma with a depressed parietal bone fracture)
- Commence regular neurological observations

If the patient deteriorates, consider a secondary cause of brain injury contributing to the primary insult. This can be a systemic cause like hypoxaemia, hypotension, hypercarbia from hypoventilation, hyponatraemia or it could be a secondary intracranial pathology such as brain oedema, raised ICP or cerebral vasospasm.

Mr Nowak has sustained a head injury, has reduced consciousness levels, focal neurological signs (left sided weakness) and signs of raised intracranial pressure (headache, vomiting, papilloedema). After stabilising him with an A to E approach, the next priority would be to urgently refer him to the neurosurgeons for definitive surgical management. In the meantime, it is vital to perform regular neurological observations to monitor for deterioration, and minimise any secondary causes of brain injury by optimising his respiratory and circulatory function. After initial assessment, the minimum frequency of initial observations for patients with a GCS of < 15 should be half-hourly for 2 hours, then hourly for 4 hours and 2-hourly thereafter. All patients must be discussed with neurosurgeons as neurological impairment is potentially reversible if the extradural haematoma is treated early. Always involve the critical care team early on – patients with deteriorating levels of consciousness should be intubated as hypocarbia and adequate oxygenation can reduce ICP rapidly.

Hand over to Mr. Smith (Neurosurgical SpR)

Situation – Hi Mr Smith, I am ____, the FY2 in A&E. I have just seen a 33 year old construction worker Mr. Nowak, who was brought in after losing consciousness following a head injury at work. He has regained consciousness but is now lethargic with left-sided weakness, a persistent headache, nausea and vomiting. A CT showed a right-sided extradural haematoma with a depressed parietal bone fracture.

Background – Mr. Nowak is normally fit and well with no medical history of note. He is not on any regular medications and has no known allergies. We are awaiting more details of the circumstances around the injury.

Assessment – His current observations are HR: 115 BP: 130/90, RR: 21 SaO$_2$: 96 % (RA) Temp: 36.9 °C. He is maintaining his airway, and is responsive to voice with a GCS of 13 (E3 V4 M6). On examination, he is drowsy and has left-sided MRC grade 3/5 weakness in both upper and lower limbs with extensor plantar reflex. There is papilloedema on fundoscopy. On full exposure, he had no other injuries of note, and there was no otorrhoea or rhinorrhoea. I have initiated regular neurological observations to monitor for any deterioration.

Recommendation – In summary Mr. Jones has a right-sided extradural haemorrhage with a depressed parietal bone fracture and signs of raised intracranial pressure. He is currently protecting his airway but I am concerned he may deteriorate. I would be grateful if you can assess him urgently. Is there anything else you would like me to do?

Head injury in brief

1. Head injuries are a common presentation in A&E. What are the criteria for performing a CT head scan?

The criteria differ between the adult and paediatric populations. A provisional written radiology report should always be available within 1 hour of the scan.

A CT scan should be performed within ONE HOUR for adults who have sustained a head injury and have any ONE of the following risk features:
- GCS <13 on initial assessment
- GCS <15 (or baseline GCS) 2 hours after injury
- Suspected open or depressed skull fracture
- Any sign of basal skull fracture (haemotypanum, 'racoon eyes', CSF otorrhoea/ rhinorrhoea, Battle's sign)
- Post-traumatic seizure
- Focal neurological deficit
- >1 episode of vomiting

A CT scan should be performed within EIGHT HOURS of injury if any of the following risk factors are present:
- Age >65 years old
- History of bleeding or clotting disorder
- Dangerous mechanism of injury
- >30 minutes of retrograde amnesia of events immediately before the head injury

2. How should patients with minor head injuries not requiring admission be managed?

All patients with any degree of head injury should be discharged with both verbal and written head injury advice. Safety-netting is key and patients must be aware of symptoms that would require them to return to A&E. They should be given the contact details of community and hospital services in case of delayed complications – some patients appear to make a rapid recovery but experience difficulties later on. Patients should also be given appropriate advice on returning to everyday activities like school/work/sports and driving.

Patients should not be discharged if there is no one suitable at home to supervise them, unless the risk of late complications is deemed negligible or suitable supervision/ follow-up arrangements have been organised.

Endocrine Emergencies

Ruslan Zinchenko

Hypoglycaemia	154
Diabetes and Diabetic Ketoacidosis (DKA)	158
Hyperosmolar Hyperglycaemic State (HHS)	162
Thyroid Storm	166
Adrenal Insufficiency	170

Case 1 – **Hypoglycaemia**

You are a Foundation Year 1 doctor working on the endocrinology and diabetes ward. A ward nurse approaches you regarding Mrs. Guptill, a 43-year-old lady with insulin dependent diabetes mellitus. She was admitted with a chest infection for IV antibiotics, and is now behaving strangely. She was given her insulin earlier and has suddenly become confused and irritable. She also appears to be shaky and is sweating profusely.

Please conduct an A to E assessment of Mrs Guptill and commence the initial management.

Latest observations:

HR: 100 BP: 129/83 RR: 21 SaO_2: 97 % (on room air) Temp: 36.9 °C ; UO: not available

Danger
It is safe to approach the patient

Response
The patient appears confused and cannot answer your questions coherently

Airway
The patient is talking, so you can assume the airway is patent.

Breathing
Look – Patient appears shaky and slightly tachypnoeaic
Feel – Normal tracheal position, chest expansion and percussion note
Listen – Normal breath sounds bilaterally
Measure – RR: 21 SaO_2: 97 % (on room air)
Treat – Move on

Circulation
Look – Patient appears sweaty and pale
Feel – Hands are warm to touch and sweaty
Listen – Normal heart sounds
Measure – HR: 100, regular BP: 129/83 UO: Temp: 36.9 °C; UO: not available
Treat – Patient has IV access, move on

Disability
AVPU – Patient is now only responsive to pain/GCS 10 (E2, V3, M5)
Capillary blood glucose – 1.9 mmol/L
Pupils/Neurology – Equal and reactive to light, reduced movement in the left limbs

---

The patient is severely hypoglycaemic and is demonstrating neurological symptoms. The hypoglycaemia should therefore be treated immediately to avoid permanent neurological sequelae. She should receive glucose and have an urgent senior review. Intravenous glucose should be used, as the patient will be unable to swallow (see Box 1).

The patient improves following intravenous glucose administration, and should now recieve a sugary drink, biscuits or a sandwich to maintain her sugars. Her capillary blood sugars will have to be frequently monitored initially.

Exposure

On full exposure, there is no evidence of bleeding or rashes and the abdomen is soft and non-tender.

Hand over the patient to Dr Patel (Endocrinology SpR)

Situation – This is Dr _____ the F1 in Endocrinology and Diabetes. I have just seen Mrs Guptill, a 43-year-old lady, who has suffered a severe hypoglycaemic episode.

Background – Mrs. Guptill is an insulin dependent diabetic, who was admitted with a chest infection. The ward nurse has asked me to review her since she has become confused and irritable following insulin administration.

Assessment – On initial assessment she appeared pale, sweaty and shaky. She was slightly tachypnoeaic but was saturating at 97 % on room air. Even though she appeared sweaty she was not pyrexic. During the assessment she became only responsive to pain, her GCS dropped to 10 and she developed left-sided weakness. Her capillary blood glucose was 1.9 mmol/L. I immediately treated this with intravenous glucose following which she markedly improved.

Recommendation – This lady has suffered a hypoglycaemic episode which has now been treated. Would you be able to review the patient and is there anything else you would like me to do?

> **Box 1. Management of Hypoglycaemia**
>
> If the patient is unable to swallow or has a low GCS, then glucose should be given intravenously (200 ml of 10 % glucose or 100 ml of 20 % glucose STAT). If there is no intravenous access (IV), administer 1mg glucagon intramuscularly whilst obtaining IV access. If the patient is able to swallow, give them a sugary drink or glucose gel. This should be followed up with more carbohydrates e.g. a sandwich.

Hypoglycaemia in brief:

1. What is the definition of hypoglycaemia?
Hypoglycaemia can be defined using the Whipple's triad, which includes:
- Symptoms of hypoglycaemia (hunger, confusion, irritability, drowsiness)
- Low blood glucose concentration (<4 mmol/L)
- Resolution of symptoms following the administration of the appropriate amount of glucose.

Symptoms and signs of hypoglycaemia do not correlate well with blood sugar levels, and vary greatly between individuals.

2. What are the causes of hypoglycaemia?
The most common causes are:
- Excessive insulin administration
- Oral hypoglycaemics (e.g. sulfonylureas).
- Alcohol (causes severe hypoglycaemia in diabetics)

Rare causes of hypoglycaemia include:
- Addison's disease
- Pituitary insufficiency
- Pancreatic tumours (insulinoma)

Case 2 – **Diabetes and Diabetic Ketoacidosis (DKA)**

You are a Foundation Year 2 doctor working in the Emergency Department. The triage nurse asks you to urgently review an 18-year-old man, Mr Ashley, who presents with nausea, vomiting and abdominal pain. He has a background of type 1 diabetes and has been complaining of polydipsia, polyuria and tiredness over the past week or so, but attributed this to the binge drinking during his Ibiza trip from which he returned yesterday. The nurse has asked you to see him because he has become less responsive.

Please conduct an A to E assessment of Mr Ashley and commence initial management.

Latest observations:

HR: 126 BP: 88/59 RR: 30 SaO$_2$: 98 % (on room air) temp: 35.6°C; UO: not available

Danger
It is safe to approach the patient

Response
The patient is responsive to pain

Airway
The airway is patent with no added sounds

Breathing
Look – Kussmaul respiration (deep, laboured breathing)
Feel – Normal tracheal position, chest expansion and percussion note
Listen – Normal breath sounds bilaterally
Measure – RR: 30 SaO$_2$: 98 % (on room air)
Treat – Move on

Circulation
Look – Pale, sweaty, sunken eyes, dry mucous membranes
Feel – Reduced skin turgor, acetone breath, and CRT 4 seconds
Listen – Normal heart sounds
Measure – HR 126, regular; BP 88/59; temp 35.6 °C UO: not available
Treat – Obtain IV access. Fluid resuscitate this patient guided by your hospital's DKA protocol and insert a urinary catheter to monitor their fluid balance.
Reassess – BP rises to 105/72 and HR slows down to 106 following commencement of fluid resuscitation.

Further Investigations:
- Perform an ECG (sinus tachycardia)
- Bloods (FBC, U&Es, LFTs, CRP, osmolality, glucose)
- Urine sample - positive for glucose and ketones

The patient may require high dependency unit admission for accurate fluid balance monitoring and rehydration.

Disability
AVPU – Patient is responsive to pain/GCS 10 (E2, V3, M5)
Capillary blood glucose – 29 mmol/L
Pupils/Neurology – equal and reactive to light, moving all four limbs

At this point you should suspect a diabetic ketoacidosis (DKA) and investigate the patient with a venous blood gas (VBG) for pH, bicarbonate, glucose, ketones, Na$^+$ and K$^+$. A blood point of care test for ketones and urine dipstick for ketones and glucose should also be done.

Once DKA is confirmed with a low pH (<7.3), hyperglycaemia and high blood ketones, you should continue fluid resuscitating the patient. An example of a fluid replacement regimen is 1 L in the first hour, 1 L over the next 2 hours, 1 L over the next 4 hours and 1 L over the next 8 hours. However, do adjust the fluids according to urine output and use local hospital guidelines. Also monitor the patient's blood potassium level, which may fall and will need replacing.

Exposure

On full exposure, there is no evidence of bleeding, rashes and the abdomen is soft and non-tender. Urine dip positive for glucose and ketones.

Hand over the patient to Dr Martin (Medical SpR):

Situation – Hello Dr Martin, my name is Dr _____ and I am the FY2 doctor in A&E. I am calling you regarding Mr Ashley, an 18 year-old man who is in DKA.

Background – He presented to A&E with nausea, vomiting and abdominal pain having returned from Ibiza yesterday. He had polydipsia, polyuria and fatigue over the past week.

Assessment – On assessment he was drowsy and only responsive to pain, with capillary blood glucose of 29 mmol/L and tachypnoea with a rate of 30. He was pale, sweaty and with dry mucous membranes. He had reduced skin turgor, a CRT of 4 seconds and I could smell acetone on his breath. His was tachycardic 126 and his BP was 92/61. These have improved following a fluid challenge of 500 ml NaCl 0.9 %. I have inserted a urinary catheter and taken some bloods. On the venous blood gas he was acidotic with a pH of 7.28, had high ketones and low bicarbonate.

Recommendation – I would like you to come and review this young man. In the mean time I will continue the rehydration regimen with 0.9 % NaCl and then start a fixed rate insulin infusion according to the hospital guidelines. Is there anything else you would like me to do?

Fixed rate insulin infusion

Please follow your local hospital guidelines when writing up an insulin infusion. However, a general principle that can be used is to dilute 50 units of soluble insulin in 50 mL of 0.9 % NaCl and set up the infusion at 0.1 units/kg/hr. It is important to keep monitoring blood glucose, ketones and bicarbonate. Blood glucose should fall by 3 mmol/L/hr, blood ketones should fall by 0.5 mmol/L/hr and venous HCO_3^- should rise by 3 mmol/L/hr. Keep monitoring the patient with frequent venous blood gases. When glucose falls below 14 mmol/l you should start a 10 % glucose infusion at 125 mL/hour. The insulin infusion can be stopped once venous pH is above 7.3, HCO_3^- is above 18 mmol/L, ketones are less than 0.3 mmol/L and the patient is eating. You should continue the patient's long acting/basal insulin throughout.

Diabetes in brief

1. How would you diagnose diabetes mellitus?
- Fasting venous glucose ≥7 mmol/L or random venous glucose ≥11.1 mmol/L with symptoms of hyperglycaemia (fatigue, weight loss, polyuria and polydipsia).
- If no symptoms of hyperglycaemia, a second confirmatory venous blood glucose sample is required, either fasting (≥7 mmol/L) or random (≥11.1 mmol/L).
- HbA1c ≥6.5 % (48 mmol/L), but it's not so useful in children with type 1 DM

2. How would you diagnose impaired glucose tolerance (IGT)?
- Fasting venous glucose <7 mmol/L
- Following an oral glucose tolerance test blood glucose is ≥7.8 mmol/L but <11.1 mmol/L

3. How would you diagnose impaired fasting glucose (IFG)?
- Venous blood glucose ≥6.1 mmol/L but <7 mmol/L

4. What are the common types of insulin?
- Fast acting insulin – **insulin aspart** or **lispro**, used at the start of a meal or straight after.
- Short acting **soluble insulin**, given 30 min before a meal or combined with a longer acting insulin e.g. **soluble insulin aspart** (30%) with **protamine-crystallised insulin aspart** 70%)
- Intermediate acting insulin – **isophane** can be taken with short acting insulin before a meal or by itself before sleep. Regulates blood sugars through out the day.
- Long acting insulin – **glargine** or **detemir**, can be injected once or twice daily. Controls blood glucose through out the day.

5. What are the common insulin regimens in type 1 diabetes?
- Twice daily regimen with premixed insulin in patients with a regular lifestyle
- Four times daily regimen with fast acting insulin before meals with a long acting insulin before bedtime.

Case 3 – **Hyperosmolar Hyperglycaemic State (HHS)**

You are a Foundation Year 2 doctor working on nights in the Emergency Department. You are asked to see Mr Barter, an 86-year-old retired lawyer with long-standing type 2 diabetes, who was brought by ambulance in a confused state. For the past week he has been excessively thirsty and has been passing large amounts of urine. His diabetes is normally poorly controlled and he suffers from recurrent UTIs.

Please conduct an A to E assessment of Mr Barter and commence the initial management.

Latest observations:
HR: 127 BP: 97/60 RR: 23 SaO$_2$: 95 % (on room air) Temp: 35.9 °C ; U/O: not available

Danger
It is safe to approach the patient

Response
The patient appears confused

Airway
The airway is patent with no added sounds

Breathing
Look – no use of accessory muscles, no central cyanosis
Feel – normal tracheal position, chest expansion and percussion note
Listen – normal breath sounds bilaterally
Measure – RR: 23 SaO$_2$: 98 % (on room air)
Treat – move on

Circulation
Look – pale, sunken eyes, dry mucous membranes
Feel – reduced skin turgor, CRT 5 seconds
Listen – normal heart sounds
Measure – HR 127, regular; BP 97/60; temp 35.9 °C U/O: not available
Treat – obtain IV access. Fluid resuscitate this patient guided by biochemical results and aim for a drop in glucose of 4-6 mmol/L/hr and a sodium drop of no more than 10 mmol/L/24hr. Insert a urinary catheter to carefully monitor the fluid balance.
Reassess – BP rises to 110/79 and HR slows down to 104 following commencement of fluid resuscitation

Further Investigations:
- Perform an ECG (sinus tachycardia)
- VBG - metabolic acidosis with severe hypernatraemia (Na$^+$158)
- Bloods (FBC,U&Es, osmolality) - Na$^+$158, osmolality 345 mmol/kg

Disability
AVPU – patient is responsive to pain/GCS 10 (E2 V3 M5)
Capillary blood glucose – 50 mmol/L
Pupils/Neurology – equal and reactive to light, moving all four limbs

At this point you should suspect either DKA or HHS. You should investigate this with a venous blood gas for pH, bicarbonate, glucose, ketones, Na^+ and K^+ and blood plasma osmolality. A urine dipstick for ketones and glucose should also be done. Hyperosmolar hyperglycaemic state will be suggested by a pH of >7.3, blood ketones <3, and osmolality of >320 mosmol/kg.

Exposure

On full exposure, there is no evidence of bleeding or rashes and the abdomen is soft and non-tender. Urine dipstick positive for nitrites and leukocytes.

Hand over the patient to Dr Moler (Medical SpR):

Situation – Hello Dr Moler, my name is Dr _____ and I am the FY2 doctor in A&E. I am calling you regarding Mr Barter, a 86 year-old man who I suspect is in hyperosmolar hyperglycaemic state as a result of a urinary tract infection.

Background – He has a long-standing history of type 2 diabetes that is poorly controlled and suffers from recurrent UTIs. For the past week he was complaining of polydipsia and polyuria.

Assessment – When I assessed him he was only responsive to pain with a GCS of 10. His airway was patent. On examination of his respiratory system he was tachypnoeaic but was saturating well at 98 % on room air. He did appear to have an overall fluid deficit with reduced central skin turgor and a CRT of 5 s. He was tachycardic at 127 and hypotensive with a BP of 97/60. I commenced appropriate fluid resuscitation as per hospital guidelines. His capillary blood glucose was 50 mmol/L which was confirmed with a venous blood gas. However he wasn't acidotic and had a blood plasma osmolality of 345 mosmol/kg and a Na^+ 158.

Recommendation – I therefore suspect this patient is in an HHS and I would like you to urgently review him. In the mean time I will continue rehydrating the patient and treat his UTI. Is there anything else you would like me to do?

Hyperosmolar hyperglycaemic state and type 2 diabetes in brief

1. How would you treat a patient who presents in HHS?
- Slow rehydration with 0.9 % NaCl over 2 days
- DVT prophylaxis with low molecular weight heparin
- Replace K^+ guided by blood K^+ concentration
- Consider insulin when the fall in glucose has plateaued with fluid therapy alone, but beware of sudden drops as these increase the risk of cerebral oedema due to intracellular fluid shifts.

2. What medications are used in the treatment of type 2 diabetes mellitus?
Commonly used medications

If diet and lifestyle measures fail – Biguanides (ie. Metformin)
- Increase insulin sensitivity and reduce weight
- Warn patients about abdominal pain, nausea and diarrhoea
- Stop metformin in acutely unwell patients with tissue hypoxia (ie. sepsis); before general anaesthesia; and in patients undergoing radiological investigations with iodine contrast

Sulfonylureas (ie. Gliclazide)
- Add if glucose control inadequate with metformin
- Stimulates insulin secretion
- Important side effects include hypoglycaemia and weight gain. May be unsuitable in overweight patients.

Insulin
- If blood glucose control still inadequate following 2 oral medications consider adding insulin.
- A long acting insulin (Glargine or Detemir) at bedtime is commonly used first line

Less commonly used medications: :

Thiazolidinediones (ie. Pioglitazone)
- Increase insulin sensitivity, and can be used instead of biguanides or sulfonylureas
- Can cause hypoglycaemia, fluid retention, fractures, deranged LFTs and increases risk of malignancy
- Avoid in patients with congestive heart failure and osteoporosis

Glucagon-like peptide (GLP) analogues (ie. Exenatide)
- Mimic incretins and stimulate insulin release whilst reducing the release of glucagon
- Can be tried instead of insulin
- Avoid in severe renal failure (eGFR <30)
- Increase the risk of developing pancreatitis

Dipeptidyl peptidase 4 (DPP-4) inhibitors (ie. Sitagliptin)
- Increase GLP concentration and therefore stimulate insulin release
- Can be used instead of insulin
- Reduce appetite and therefore may be tried in the obese
- Avoid in renal failure (eGFR <50)
- Increase the risk of developing pancreatitis

Case 4 – **Thyroid Storm**

You are a Foundation Year 1 doctor covering the medical wards at night. Mrs Volvitt, a 46-year-old lady was admitted yesterday for radioiodine treatment of medication resistant Grave's disease. She received her first dose of radioiodine this afternoon. An endocrinology ward bleeps you in the middle of the night to tell you that Mrs Volvitt is feeling extremely unwell and asks for your help urgently.

Please conduct an A to E assessment of Mrs Volvitt and commence the initial management.

Latest observations:

HR: 160 BP: 136/87 RR: 28 SaO$_2$: 96 % (on room air) Temp: 39.0 °C; U/O: not available

Danger

It is safe to approach the patient

Response

The patient appears agitated and confused

Airway

The patient is talking to you so you assume the airway is patent.

Breathing

Look – Normal breathing effort, no central cyanosis
Feel – Normal tracheal position, however you feel a soft, smooth mass overlying it
Listen – Normal breath sounds bilaterally
Measure – RR: 28 SaO_2: 96 % (on room air)
Treat – Move on

Circulation

Look – Agitated, sweaty
Feel – Hot to touch, CRT <2 seconds
Listen – Flow murmur
Measure – HR 160, irregularly irregular; BP 136/87; temp 39.0 °C U/O: N/A
Treat – Obtain IV access. Give paracetamol for pyrexia and a beta-blocker (e.g. propranolol) to rate control and counteract the peripheral effects of thyroid hormones. Diltiazem can be used if beta-blockers are contraindicated. Ask for help at this point
Reassess – HR slows down to 120 following propranolol, temperature 37.5 °C

Further investigations
- Perform an ECG (fast atrial fibrillation)
- Continuous BP monitoring (patient at risk of high output heart failure)
- Blood (FBC, U&Es, LFTs, CRP, blood cultures)
- Blood (TSH, free T_4, free T_3)

Do not wait for blood results since urgent treatment is needed. The patient is at risk of cardiovascular collapse and will have to be managed in a high dependency unit. You should contact the Endocrinology SpR/Medical SpR. For further management of a thyroid storm see Box 1.

Disability

AVPU – Patient is alert/GCS 14 (E4, V4, M6)
Capillary blood glucose – 3.9 mmol/L
Pupils – equal and reactive to light

Exposure

On full exposure the patient is sweaty and hot to touch. There is no evidence of bleeding, rashes and the abdomen is soft and non-tender.

Hand over the patient to Dr Boer (Medical SpR):

Situation – Hello Dr Boer, my name is Dr _____ and I am the FY1 doctor covering the medical wards. I am calling you regarding Mrs Volvitt, a 46-year-old woman who I suspect is having a thyroid storm.

Background – She was admitted yesterday for radioiodine treatment of medication resistant Grave's disease. She received her first dose of radioiodine this afternoon.

Assessment – When I saw her she appeared agitated and confused. She was also sweaty and hot to touch. She had a soft smooth mass in her anterior neck. Her respiratory examination was unremarkable apart from mild tachypnoea. She was tachycardic at 160 bpm with an irregularly irregular rhythm. However, she was haemodynamically stable with a BP of 136/87. She was also pyrexic with a temperature of 39.0 °C. An ECG demonstrated fast atrial fibrillation. She is now on continuous cardiac monitoring and I have sent off some routine bloods including FBC and U&Es as well as thyroid function tests. I have given her paracetamol 1 g IV for pyrexia and 40mg of propranolol. She responded to both of the drugs and her temperature now is 37.5°C and her HR is 120.

Recommendation – I suspect she is having a thyroid storm following radioiodine treatment. I would like you to come and review her urgently as I think she is at risk of cardiovascular collapse. Is there anything you would like me to do in the meantime?

> **Box 1. Management of a thyroid storm**
>
> - This should be done by a specialist.
> - Propranolol may be used to counteract the peripheral effects of thyroid hormones. If propranolol is contraindicated eg asthma or heart failure, then diltiazem may be used.
> - Digoxin may also be used to reduce the tachycardia.
> - Anti-thyroid drugs (ie. carbimazole) are then used to reduce the production of T_3 & T_4.
> - Hydrocortisone or dexamethasone may be used to reduce peripheral conversion of T_4 to T_3.
> - Paracetamol is used for pyrexia.
> - IV fluids are given if the patient is dehydrated.

Thyrotoxicosis in brief

1. What would thyroid function tests demonstrate in thyrotoxicosis?
Thyroid stimulating hormone (TSH) would be suppressed, whereas T_3 and T_4 would be increased.

2. What are the causes of thyrotoxicosis?
- Grave's disease
- Toxic multinodular goiter
- Toxic adenoma
- Thyroid cancer (follicular carcinoma)
- Viral thyroiditis (de Quervain's thyroiditis)
- Drugs (iodine, levothyroxine, amiodarone, lithium)

3. What can trigger a thyroid storm?
- Abrupt withdrawal of anti-thyroid medication
- Radioiodine
- Stressors (sepsis, trauma, myocardial infarction)

Case 5 – **Adrenal Insufficiency**

You are a Foundation Year 1 doctor covering the general medicine wards. In the middle of the night you are bleeped by one of the ward nurses regarding Ms Burton, a 25-year-old female, who was admitted with community acquired pneumonia 2 days ago. She has a history of poorly controlled asthma and normally takes high dose oral prednisolone. The nurse tells you that she was slightly confused in the afternoon but has now become less responsive.

Please conduct an A to E assessment of Ms Burton and commence the initial management.

Latest observations:

HR: 131 BP: 89/58 RR: 23 SaO_2: 97 % (on room air) temp: 36.7°C; UO: not available

Danger

It is safe to approach the patient

Response

The patient is responsive to your voice with groans

Airway

The patient is groaning, so you can assume the airway is patent.

Breathing

Look – normal breathing effort, not central cyanosis or accessory muscle use
Feel – normal tracheal position, chest expansion and percussion note
Listen – normal breath sounds bilaterally
Measure – RR: 23 SaO_2: 97 % (on room air)
Treat – move on

Circulation

Look – pale
Feel – cold extremities, weak peripheral pulses, CRT = 6 seconds
Listen – normal heart sounds
Measure – HR 131, regular; BP 89/58; temp 36.7 °C UO: 250 ml over 12 hours
Treat – IV NaCl 0.9 % 500 ml fluids challenge STAT. Repeat if necessary up to 2000 mL.
Reassess – BP rises to 100/73 and HR slows down to 110 following the fluid challenge.

Further Investigations:
- Perform an ECG - sinus tachycardia
- Perform a VBG - hyperkalaemia and hyponatraemia
- Bloods (FBC, U&Es) - confirms hyperkalaemia with hyponatraemia
- Consider testing blood cortisol

It would be appropriate to ask for senior help at this point, as the patient is clearly unwell. The likely diagnosis is an Addisonian crisis because the patient hasn't received her usual steroids. You should therefore contact the medical registrar on call, and give IV hydrocortisone.

Disability

AVPU – Patient is responsive to voice/GCS 12 (E3, V4, M5)
Capillary blood glucose – 2.3 mmol/L
Pupils – equal and reactive to light

You should treat this patient's hypoglycaemia with intravenous glucose.

Exposure

The abdomen is soft and non-tender. There are no rashes.

Hand over the patient to Dr Smith (Medical SpR):

Situation – Hello Dr Smith, my name is Dr _____ and I am the FY1 doctor covering the general medicine wards. I am calling you regarding Ms Burton, a 25 year-old lady who I suspect is having an Addisonian crisis.

Background – She was admitted 2 days ago with a community acquired pneumonia. She also has poorly controlled asthma for which she is on long-term oral steroids.

Assessment – On assessment she was responsive to voice with a GCS of 12. She was slightly tachypnoeaic but was saturating well on room air. She was pale with cold extremities and weak pulses. Her CRT was 6 seconds. She was tachycardic at 131 bpm and hypotensive with a BP of 89/58. I gave her a fluid challenge to which she has responded and 100 mg of IV hydrocortisone. I also corrected her hypoglycaemia of 2.3 mmol/l with intravenous glucose. A VBG demonstrated hyperkalaemia and hyponatraemia, which was confirmed on a laboratory blood test. I have also sent off blood cortisol levels.

Recommendation – I would like you to come and review this young woman urgently as I suspect she is having an Addisonian crisis due to inappropriate steroid replacement therapy. Is there anything else you would like me to do in the meantime?

Adrenal insufficiency in brief

1. What is the pathophysiology of adrenal insufficiency?
Primary adrenal insufficiency results from the destruction of the adrenal cortex, which leads to the decreased production of mainly mineralocorticoids (aldosterone) and glucocorticoids (cortisol). However, deficiency of dehydroepiandrosterone (DHEAS) can also occur.

Secondary adrenal insufficiency results from the disruption of the hypothalamic-pituitary-adrenal axis leading to a reduction of ACTH.

2. What are the causes of adrenal insufficiency?
Primary adrenal insufficiency:
- Autoimmune destruction (commonest in the UK)
- Tuberculosis (commonest worldwide)
- Adrenal metastasis
- Adrenal haemorrhage (warfarin, Waterhouse-Friderichsen syndrome, antiphospholipid syndrome)
- Infections (meningicoccus, histoplasmosis, HIV)
- Drugs (ketoconazole)
- Congenital adrenal hyperplasia

Secondary adrenal insufficiency:
- Iatrogenic (long-term steroids)
- CNS disease affecting the hypothalamus or the pituitary gland

3. What laboratory tests should be considered in the diagnosis of adrenal insufficiency?
- Electrolytes – low Na^+ and high K^+ due to mineralocorticoid deficiency
- Glucose – low glucose due to glucocorticoid deficiency
- Short Synacthen® test (ACTH stimulation test): measure serum cortisol 30 min after ACTH administration - confirms adrenal insufficiency.

4. How would you treat a patient with adrenal insufficiency?
- Advise against suddenly stopping steroids
- Increase steroid dose during febrile illness or surgery
- Hydrocortisone in divided doses (2/3 of the dose in the morning and 1/3 in the afternoon) and fludrocortisone

5. What can trigger an Addisonian crisis?
- Severe illness
- Surgery, trauma
- Abrupt withdrawal of steroids

Electrolyte Emergencies
Ruslan Zinchenko

Acute Kidney Injury and Hyperkalaemia	176
Hyponatraemia	182

Case 1 – Acute Kidney Injury and Hyperkalaemia

You are a Foundation Year 1 doctor working on the care of the elderly ward. Mrs Shelton, an 83 year-old lady was admitted yesterday with urinary tract sepsis. Prior to admission she has spent several days on the floor, unable to get up following a fall, until she was discovered by one of her carers. Following the morning ward round you check up on her blood tests and discover that her K$^+$ is 7.1 mmol/L and she has acute kidney injury.

Please conduct an A to E assessment of Mrs Shelton and commence the initial management.

Latest observations:

HR: 115 BP: 90/60 RR: 30 SaO$_2$: 96 % (on room air) temp: 37.8 °C; U/O: 100 ml over 12 hours

Danger
It is safe to approach the patient

Response
The patient is confused, but looks at you when you introduce yourself

Airway
The patient is talking; the airway is patent with no added sounds

Breathing
Look – normal respiration with no central cyanosis
Feel – normal tracheal position, chest expansion and percussion note
Listen – normal breath sounds bilaterally
Measure – RR: 30 SaO$_2$: 96 % (on room air)
Treat – move on

Circulation
Look – JVP non-visible, sunken eyes, dry mucous membranes
Feel – reduced skin turgor, CRT 4 seconds
Listen – normal heart sounds
Measure – HR 115 irregularly irregular; BP 90/60; temp 37.8 °C U/O: 100 ml over 12 hours
Treat – resuscitate with IV fluids (250mL boluses), guided by patient's fluid balance. Give calcium gluconate, insulin-glucose infusion and consider nebulised salbutamol.
Reassess – BP rises to 110/80 and HR slows down to 100. Repeat K$^+$ 6.0 mmol/L

Further Investigations:
- ECG - bradycardia, tall tented T-waves, absent P-waves, wide QRS complexes
- Place the patient on a cardiac monitor
- Urgently perform a VBG to confirm the raised K$^+$
- Repeat bloods (FBC, U&E, CK) to re-assess her renal function and look for rhabdomyolysis

---

This patient demonstrates ECG changes associated with hyperkalaemia, which could lead to VT/VF and cardiac arrest. Urgent treatment is therefore required. Refer to Box 1 for further details on the acute management of hyperkalaemia.

Disability

AVPU – Patient is responsive to voice/GCS12 (E3 V4 M5)
Capillary blood glucose – 8.6 mmol/L
Pupils – equal and reactive to light

Exposure

On full exposure, there is no evidence of bleeding or rashes and the adomenis soft and non-tender. You flush the urinary catheter to ensure it's working.

> Review the patient's drug chart and stop any nephrotoxic drugs and those that could be contributing to the hyperkalaemia.

Hand over the patient to Dr Medway (Care of the Elderly SpR):

Situation – Hello Dr Medway my name is Dr_____ and I am the FY1 doctor in care of the elderly. I am calling you regarding Mrs Shelton, an 83 year-old lady who is in AKI and has severe hyperkalaemia of 7.1 mmol/L with ECG changes.

Background – She was admitted yesterday with urinary tract sepsis having spent several days on the floor until being discovered by her carers.

Assessment – On examination she was confused with a GCS of 12. Her respiratory examination was normal. However, she was clinically dehydrated with dry mucous membranes, reduced skin turgor and a CRT of 4 s. She was tachycardic at 115 bmp with an irregularly irregular rate and hypotensive with a BP of 90/60. She was also pyrexic at 37.8 °C and had a reduced UO of 100 ml over 12 hours. I gave her a fluid challenge to which she has responded and her BP rose to 110/80 whilst her HR went down to 100. I also gave her calcium gluconate and started an insulin infusion. I have also sent off repeat blood tests to reassess her renal function and to look for rhabdomyolysis.

Recommendation – I would like you to come and review this elderly lady. Is there anything else you would like me to do in the meantime?

> **Box 1. Acute management of hyperkalaemia**
>
> - Eliminate the source of hyperkalaemia – in this lady acute kidney injury should be aggressively treated with IV fluids.
> - 10 mL of 10 % calcium gluconate to stabilise the cardiac membrane if ECG changes are present. Calcium chloride may be used if there is haemodynamic compromise. The protective effect starts within minutes but is short-lived and the treatment should therefore be repeated after 5 minutes. This will not lower the serum K^+ levels.
> - To drive the K^+ intracellularly, beta-adrenergic agonists (5mg nebulised salbutamol) or an insulin-glucose infusion (10 units in 50 ml of 50 % glucose) can be used. These measures start working within 15 minutes and can generally last up to 2 hours giving you valuable time.
> - Further management gets rid of excessive K^+ in the body and includes diuretic therapy with furosemide.
> - In refractory hyperkalaemia hemodialysis may be required.

Acute kidney injury in brief

1. What are the causes of AKI?

Pre-renal – due to renal hypoperfusion:
- Hypotension (hypovolaemia, sepsis)
- Renal artery stenosis, angiotensin converting enzyme (ACE) inhibitors

Renal - due to renal tissue damage:
- Acute tubular necrosis (aminoglycosides, rhabdomyolysis, myeloma)
- Glomerular disease (glomerulonephritides, SLE)
- Interstitial nephritis (pyelonephritis, penicillins, NSAIDs)
- Renal vascular disease (vasculitis, malignant hypertension, haemolytic uraemic syndrome)

Post-renal – occlusion of the urinary tract:
- Extrinsic (pelvic/abdominal malignancy, retroperitoneal fibrosis)
- Mural (transitional cell carcinoma, strictures)
- Luminal (stones, sloughed renal papillae)

2. How do you classify acute kidney injury?

The KDIGO classification is frequently used.

STAGE	SERUM CREATININE	URINE OUTPUT
1	Increase >26 µmol/L in 48 h OR Increase of >1.5 x baseline	<0.5 mL/kg/h for more than 6 hours
2	Increase of 2 – 2.9 x baseline	<0.5 mL/kg/h for more than 12 hours
3	Increase of >3 x baseline OR >354 µmol/L OR started on dialysis	<0.3 mL/kg/h for more than 24 hours or anuria for 12 hours

3. What are the indications for dialysis in acute kidney injury?
- Uraemic encephalopathy or pericarditis
- Hyperkalaemia (K^+ >7 mmol/L) resistant to medical treatment
- Pulmonary oedema resistant to medical treatment
- Severe metabolic acidosis (pH <7.2 or Base excess <-10)
- Drug overdose (BLEST: Barbiturates, Lithium, Ethylene Glycol, Salicylates, Theophylline)

Case 2 – **Hyponatraemia**

You are a Foundation Year 1 doctor working in the Acute Medical Unit. Ms Cassiobury, a 28-year-old lady was admitted to your unit earlier that day with severe diarrhoea and vomiting. You are asked by one of the nurses to urgently review her as she has initially become confused and is now less responsive. Earlier that day she was complaining of a headache and was rather irritable.

Please conduct an A to E assessment of Ms Cassiobury and commence the initial management.

Latest observations:
HR: 115 BP: 106/75 RR: 19 SaO_2: 98 % (RA) temp: 36.8 °C; U/O: 200 ml over 8 hours

Danger
It is safe to approach the patient

Response
The patient is responsive to pain

Airway
The airway is patent with no added sounds

Breathing
Look – normal respiratory effort
Feel – normal tracheal position, chest expansion and percussion note
Listen – normal breath sounds bilaterally
Measure – RR: 19 SaO$_2$: 98 % (on room air)
Treat – move on

Circulation
Look – sunken eyes, dry mucous membranes; you notice that the patient's cannula, through which the rehydration fluids were running, has come out.
Feel – reduced skin turgor, CRT 3 seconds
Listen – normal heart sounds
Measure – HR 115, regular; BP 106/75; temp 36.8 °C U/O: 200 ml over 8 hours (looks dark)
Treat – obtain access. Restart rehydration and maintenance fluids as per patient's team instructions
Reassess – the patient's clinical status does not improve

Further Investigations:
- Perform an ECG – sinus tachycardia
- Morning U&Es: Na$^+$ 117, K$^+$ 4.8, Ur 10, Cr 110
- Test urine Na$^+$ (17 mmol/L)

The patient has severe hyponatraemia and requires cautious rehydration (see Box 1).
This is frequently a complex task and therefore it would be appropriate to ask for help in the management of this patient from your seniors.

Disability

AVPU – Patient is responsive to pain/GCS 10 (E2, V3, M5)
Capillary blood glucose – 3.8 mmol/L
Pupils – equal and reactive to light

Exposure

As you are about to expose Ms Cassiobury, she begins to fit. It would be appropriate to perform the A to E assessment all over again to make sure the patient is maintaining her airway and give the patient high flow oxygen (10–15 L via a non re-breathe mask)

> You should ask for senior help immediately since managing hyponatraemia induced seizures is beyond the level of competence of a foundation year doctor.

Hand over the patient to Dr Mayo (Acute Medicine SpR):

Situation – Hello Dr Mayo, my name is Dr _____ and I am the FY1 doctor in AMU. I am calling you regarding Ms Cassiobury, a 28 year-old lady with severe hyponatraemia who has just suffered a seizure.

Background – She was admitted earlier in the day with severe diarrhoea and vomiting for IV rehydration. The nurses told me that in the last few hours she was irritable and was complaining of a headache.

Assessment – On assessment she was drowsy and only responsive to pain with a GCS of 10. Her respiratory examination was normal. However she had dry mucous membranes and reduced skin turgor. Her CRT was 3 seconds. She was tachycardic and an ECG showed sinus tachycardia. Her BP was 106/75 and she has only passed 200 ml of urine over 8 hours, which was dark in colour. Her recent bloods test demonstrated severe hyponatraemia with a Na^+ 117 and dehydration. As I was examining her she began to fit. I ensured that she was maintaining her airway and put her on high flow oxygen.

Recommendation – I need your help immediately. Is there anything else you would like me to do?

> **Box 1. Management of acute symptomatic hyponatraemia**
>
> Patients with acute symptomatic hyponatraemia should be cautiously rehydrated with 0.9 % NaCl. However, it is important not to correct blood sodium quickly as this may lead to central pontine myelinolysis (CPM) which frequently results in irreversible demyelination of the pons. Patients with CPM present with confusion, pseudobulbar palsy, paraparesis, quadraparesis or coma.
>
> Serum Na$^+$ should be corrected at a maximum rate 10–15 mmol/L per day. More rapid correction should only be done in ITU settings under close supervision. If the patient becomes fluid overloaded then furosemide may be used.
>
> Patients with hyponatraemia induced seizures and coma should be managed in ITU. These patients can be rehydrated with hypertonic (1.8 %) NaCl but only under expert supervision. The target plasma Na$^+$ should be approximately 125 mmol/L.

Hyponatraemia in brief

1. What are the causes of hyponatraemia?
A good way to divide the causes of hyponatraemia is to look at the patient's fluid status which should be assessed clinically:
- Fluid deplete
- Normal fluid balance
- Fluid overloaded

Fluid deplete

These patients should have their urinary Na$^+$ checked.

Urinary Na$^+$ >20 mmol/L:
- Diuretic overuse
- Diuresis of renal disease
- Addison's disease
- Hyperglycaemia (diabetes mellitus)

Urinary Na⁺ <20 mmol/L:
- Diarrhoea and vomiting
- Burns
- Fistulae
- Small bowel obstruction
- Overheating
- Cystic fibrosis

Normal fluid balance:
- SIADH (syndrome of inappropriate antidiuretic hormone secretion)
- Severe hypothyroidism
- Glucocorticoid deficiency

Fluid overloaded:
- Congestive cardiac failure
- Renal failure
- Nephrotic syndrome
- Liver cirrhosis

2. What drugs can be used to treat resistant hyponatraemia?
Vaptans (e.g. tolvaptan), are vasopressor receptor antagonists that act on the vasopressin type 2 receptors in the collecting duct of the nephron. They can be used in hyponatraemia, which fails to respond to 0.9 % NaCl. These drugs increase the renal excretion of water whilst preserving Na⁺ and K⁺. They are effective in treating patients with fluid overload and normal fluid balance.

Alternatively demeclocycline, an antibiotic, may be given, however it is rarely used because of its side effect profile (nausea, vomiting, diarrhoea, hepatotoxicity, photosensitivity).

3. What causes SIADH?
- Major surgery and trauma
- Malignancy (small-cell lung cancer, lymphoma)
- Brain pathology (stroke, infection, injury)
- Chest pathology (infection, malignancy)
- Drugs (opiates, SSRIs esp. fluoxetine)

This is a very common cause of hyponatraemia in hospital inpatients and is usually managed with fluid restriction and vaptans.

Oncological Emergencies

Brian Chua and Ruslan Zinchenko

Neutropenic Sepsis	190
Acute Spinal Cord Compression	194
Acute Hypercalcaemia	198
Tumour Lysis Syndrome	204

Case 1 – **Neutropenic Sepsis**

You are a Foundation Year 1 doctor working on the haematology ward. You are asked to see Mr. Thomson, a 30-year-old man, who has become generally unwell overnight with a fever, sore throat and a non-productive cough. He had been started on inpatient chemotherapy the week before for his non-Hodgkin's lymphoma.

Please perform an A to E assessment of Mr Thomson and commence the initial management.

Latest observations:
HR: 130 BP: 80/50 RR: 22 SaO$_2$: 95 % (room air) Temp: 39.0 °C U/O: N/A

Danger
It is safe to approach the patient

Response
The patient is drowsy and responsive to voice

Airway
Mr. Thomson is mumbling some words. His airway is patent.

Breathing
Look – Sitting upright, tachypnoeic
Feel – Symmetrical chest expansion; chest is resonant to percussion bilaterally
Listen – Vesicular breath sounds bilaterally
Measure – RR 22 SaO_2 95 % (RA)
Treat – No treatment necessary at present

Further investigations:
- Consider a chest XR

Circulation
Look – Looks cachectic and pale with conjunctival pallor, Hickman line in situ
Feel – Regular, low volume pulse. Hot peripheries. No oedema.
Listen – Heart sounds normal.
Measure – HR 130; BP 80/50; Temp: 39.0 °C, U/O: NA
Treat – Obtain IV access, fluid resuscitate this patient (e.g. boluses of 500 mL of crystalloid), give paracetamol 1 g as the patient is pyrexial. Insert a urinary catheter.
Reassess – There is slight haemodynamic improvement: HR 110, BP 100/60. Further fluid resuscitation is required.

Further investigations:
- Bloods (FBC, U&E, LFT, CRP)
- Cultures (blood, urine and throat)
- VBG (pH 7.25, lactate 5.0 mmol/L, bicarbonate 16.0 mmol/L)

Disability

AVPU – responsive to voice/GCS 13 (E3, V4, M6)
Glucose – 4.8 mmol/L
Pupils/neurology – Equal and reactive to light, moving all 4 limbs

Exposure

Patient has a mobile, rubbery, non-tender lump situated in the right submandibular region. It is well demarcated with a smooth surface and is non-pulsatile. You also notice multiple bruises on all his limbs.

> At this point you should suspect neutropenic sepsis and, having taken blood cultures, you should immediately commence broad-spectrum antibiotics. Antibiotics such as meropenem, cefepime or ceftazidime may be suitable.
>
> In view of widespread bruising and an underlying malignancy, clotting studies should also be carried out (INR & APTT).

Hand over the patient to Dr Jones (Acute Oncology SpR)

Situation - My name is Dr_____ and I an FY1 in haematology. I have just seen Mr. Thomson who I suspect has neutropenic sepsis.

Background – Mr. Thomson has non-Hodgkins lymphoma and has been commenced on chemotherapy one week ago. Earlier today he started feeling generally unwell complaining of a sore throat and a dry cough.

Assessment – On initial assessment, Mr. Thomson was drowsy but responsive to voice. He was haemodynamically compromised, running a tachycardia of 130 and had a BP of 80/50. This has improved following fluid resuscitation. He is also pyrexic at 39.0 °C and I have given him paracetamol. He has lactic acidosis on his VBG.

On further examination, he looked cachectic, pale and had multiple bruises. He also has a mobile, non-tender, well-demarcated lump with a smooth surface along his right submandibular region.

I suspect he has neutropenic sepsis secondary to his chemotherapy. I have sent off a set of bloods as well as blood, urine and throat cultures. I have also started him on meropenem to cover for a broad variety of organisms.

Recommendation – I would really appreciate it if you could urgently review this patient. In the meantime, is there anything you would like me to do?

Neutropenic sepsis in brief

1. What is neutropenic sepsis?
The normal range for neutrophils is 2.5 – 7.5 x 10^9/L. Neutropenia refers to a low neutrophil count. Neutropenic sepsis is defined as neutropenia of <0.5 x 10^9/L and a temperature of >38 °C or >37.5 °C on two separate occasions at least 1 hour apart, or other clinical signs of sepsis.

Neutropenic sepsis typically presents 7 days after treatment and is more common in malignancies with high cell turnover such as leukaemia and lymphoma.

2. What is the pathophysiology and aetiology of neutropenic sepsis?
Neutrophils are granulocytes, which originate from the line of myeloblasts, and form part of the innate immunity. They are particularly active against bacteria, and engulf these microorganisms via phagocytosis. Hence, a low neutrophil level makes you susceptible to bacterial infections.

There are a variety of conditions, which may result in a low neutrophil count. This can be a result of increased destruction of neutrophils due to infections such as malaria and hypersplenism. It can also occur if the production of neutrophils is affected, which can occur in blood malignancies such as leukaemia and lymphoma, chemo-radiotherapy for any cancer, aplastic anaemia and certain drugs such as gold and penicillamine.

3. How should patients with neutropenic sepsis be managed?
A patient with a suspected neutropenic sepsis is an acute oncological emergency and should be treated without delay. Having said that, it is important to identify the source of infection and the causative organism in these patients, so that the appropriate antimicrobial therapy can be given.

Therefore one should do urine, sputum, mouth/rectal/wound/Hickman line swabs and blood cultures as well as a chest radiograph. However, these should be done as soon as possible after the patient's presentation and should not delay the commencement of broad-spectrum antibiotics. Patients with significant neutropenia should be placed in isolation to reduce the risk of cross-infections and should be referred to the acute oncology service early on.

Each hospital will have its own guidelines for the treatment of neutropenic sepsis, and if in doubt you should discuss the patients with the on call microbiology team. In general the treatment should cover a broad spectrum of gram-positive and negative microorganisms. Therefore a suitable broad-spectrum regimen is IV piperacillin with tazobactam (Tazocin) or meropenem. Further antibiotics may be required depending on the source of the infection. For example, one might consider covering for Staphylococcus aureus if the suspected source of infection is from a central line.

Case 2 – **Acute Spinal Cord Compression**

You are a Foundation Year 2 doctor working nights in A&E. You have been asked to see a 72-year-old man, Mr. White, who presents with severe back pain and weakness in both of his lower limbs. He also has trouble passing urine and opening his bowels. He is known to have advanced metastatic prostate cancer.

Please perform an A to E assessment of Mr White and commence the initial management.

Latest observations:

HR: 98 BP: 115/76 RR: 18 SaO_2: 100 % (RA) Temp: 37.0 °C UO: N/A

Danger
It is safe to approach the patient

Response
Mr White is alert and responsive

Airway
Mr. White is responding in complete sentences, it is safe to assume that his airway is patent.

Breathing
Normal respiratory assessment

Circulation
Normal cardiovascular assessment

> If Mr. White has difficulties emptying his bladder, you should consider performing an ultrasound scan of the bladder to assess for any urinary retention and insert a catheter if necessary.

Disability
AVPU – Patient is alert and responsive/GCS 15
Glucose – 5.0 mmol/L
Pupils – equal and reactive to light

Since the patient presents with focal neurological deficits, it is essential to perform a full neurological examination at this point to assess the extent of the pathology. For the purpose of this exercise, only the findings of the lower limb examination will be presented but one should also examine upper limbs and the cranial nerves. .

Lower limb neurological examination

Inspection – No deformities, obvious muscle wasting or asymmetry, fasciculations or scars
Tone – Bilateral hypertonia
Power – Reduced power across all myotomes (MRC 2/5)
Coordination – impaired due to widespread weakness
Reflexes – Brisk knee (L3/L4) and ankle (S1/S2) reflexes; upgoing plantars (+ve "Babinski sign").
Sensation – Reduced sensation across all dermatomes bilaterally and the perineal area.

The clinical findings clearly point to an upper motor neuron lesion. The patient should urgently have an MRI of the spinal cord. This shows metastatic bony compression of the lumbar spinal cord (L1-2). This patient should be commenced on IV steroids (dexamethasone or methylprednisolone) and referred to the neurosurgical team for consideration of urgent decompression.

Further investigations:
- Bloods (FBC, U&E, clotting, bone profile, G&S)

Exposure

On full exposure, there is no evidence of bleeding or rashes and the abdomen is soft and non-tender. The patient will require analgesia for pain.

Hand over the patient to Mr Barret (Neurosurgical SpR)

Situation – Hello, my name is Dr_____ and I am an FY2 in A&E. I have just seen Mr. White who I suspect has acute spinal cord compression.

Background – Mr. White presented with bilateral leg weakness and is known to have advanced metastatic prostate cancer. He has also been complaining of severe back pain and inability to pass urine and open his bowels.

Assessment – On examination, Mr. White appeared well and his respiratory and cardiovascular examinations were unremarkable. However, on neurological examination of his lower limbs he had signs of an upper motor neuron lesion. The MRI of his spine showed bilateral metastatic compression of the lumbar spinal cord (L1-2). The patient has now been given 4mg of IV dexamethasone.

Recommendation – I would like you to come and review this patient for consideration of an urgent decompression surgery. In the meantime, is there anything else you would like me to do?

Spinal cord compression in brief

1. How can you clinically differentiate between acute spinal cord compression and acute cauda equina/conus medullaris lesions?

Patients with acute compression of the spinal cord present with increased spasticity and hyper-reflexia. However, do remember that reflexes may be reduced in acute spinal cord injury as a result of the spinal shock syndrome. The precise neurological findings will depend on the location of the affected segment of the spinal cord. If there is involvement of the cauda equina or conus medullaris, patients have a flaccid paralysis of the lower limbs and are areflexic.

2. What are the common causes of acute spinal cord compression and cauda equina/conus medullaris lesions?

- Metastatic disease, commonly from prostate, breast, lung, thyroid and renal malignancies
- Trauma
- Vertebral disc prolapse
- Infection leading to an epidural abscess
- Haematoma in anti-coagulated patients

3. How should patients with acute spinal cord compression be managed?

Time is critical in these patients, as the earlier the surgical spinal decompression is carried out, the higher the chances of regaining previous levels of neurological function. Therefore patients with a suspected compression of the spinal cord should have urgent MR imaging of the spine and commenced on IV dexamethasone or methylprednisolone. In patients with severe pain, analgesia should also be commenced.

Once the diagnosis has been confirmed on imaging, the patient should be referred to the neurosurgical team for consideration of spinal cord decompression surgery. If the patient is not a suitable candidate for surgery, then targeted radiotherapy should be considered instead.

Case 3 – **Acute Hypercalcaemia**

You are a Foundation Year 1 doctor working on the Acute Medical Unit. Your registrar has asked you to clerk in an 83 year-old gentleman, Stanley Burman, who was brought into A&E by the ambulance crew with confusion and being "off his legs". He is known to have multiple myeloma and is under the hospital oncology service. For the past several days he has been passing large amounts of urine. Prior to seeing the patient you look through the bloods ordered by A&E and notice that the adjusted serum Ca^{2+} is 3.8 mmol/L.

Please perform an A to E assessment of Mr Burman and commence the initial management.

Latest observations:

HR: 100 BP: 90/60 RR: 16 SaO_2: 98 % (RA) Temp: 36.5 °C UO: 100 mL dark urine

Danger
It is safe to approach the patient

Response
Mr Burman is responsive to voice, but appears confused

Airway
Mr Burman is mumbling words, it is safe to assume the airway is patent

Breathing
Look – lying flat, no signs of cyanosis or use of accessory muscles
Feel – symmetrical chest expansion; chest is resonant to percussion bilaterally
Listen – vesicular breath sounds bilaterally
Measure – RR 16 SaO_2 98 % (room air)
Treat – no treatment necessary at present, monitor for any deterioration

Circulation
Look – dry mucous membranes, looks cachectic and pale with conjunctival pallor
Feel – regular, low volume pulse, reduced skin turgor
Listen – heart sounds normal
Measure – HR 100; BP 90/60; Temp: 36.5 °C, U/O: 100 mL of dark urine
Treat – obtain IV access, commence fluid resuscitation (e.g. fluid boluses of 500 mL 0.9 % NaCl)
Reassess – There is haemodynamic improvement: HR 90, BP 100/70, however further fluid therapy (see Box 1) and medical management (see Box 2) will be required.

Further investigations:
- ECG – shortened QT interval
- Place the patient on a cardiac monitor

This patient is showing ECG changes as a result of severe hypercalcaemia and is at risk of a cardiac arrest. He will therefore require continuous cardiac monitoring until the hypercalcaemia has resolved.

> **Box 1. Fluid therapy in hypercalcaemia**
>
> Since this patient is known to have severe hypercalcaemia, appears to be clinically dehydrated, and is showing ECG changes consistent with hypercalcaemia, the first step in his management will be appropriate fluid resuscitation. Several litres of 0.9 % saline may be required and rate of fluid administration should be approximately between 250 – 500 mL/hour. However this will depend on the volume status of the patient, his cardiac and renal function. Therefore, fluids should be adjusted according to the urinary output. The saline will treat the dehydration, which occurs as a result of secondary nephrogenic diabetes insipidus caused by the high serum calcium and will promote the urinary excretion of calcium.

Disability

AVPU – Patient is responsive to voice/GCS 13 (E3, V4, M6)
Glucose – 9.1 mmol/L
Pupils/neurology – equal and reactive to light, moving all four limbs

Exposure

There are no rashes and the abdomen is soft and non-tender.

> **Box 2. Medical management of hypercalcaemia**
>
> Once patients with malignancy-associated hypercalcaemia have been rehydrated, they are best-treated with intravenous bisphosphonates, which act on osteoclasts to reduce bone resorption. Either pamidronate or zoledronate can be given as a single dose. They take between 2 – 4 days to reach therapeutic effect and should therefore be administered early on.
>
> Calcitonin has a quicker onset of action and also interferes with osteoclastic bone resorption. It may be given in the short-term, to transiently lower the serum calcium, whilst waiting for the bisphosphonates to start acting. Furosemide may be given to increase the renal excretion of calcium. However, it should be used cautiously to avoid further fluid depletion, and should be introduced once the patient has been fully rehydrated. All medications, which may increase serum calcium levels (thiazides, vitamin D etc.) should be stopped. Ultimately, the treatment of the underlying malignancy will treat the hypercalcaemia in the long-term.

Hand over the patient to Dr Jones (Acute oncology SpR)

Situation – Hello, My name is Dr_____ and I am the AMU FY1. I am calling you regarding Mr Burman, an 83 year-old man with severe hypercalcaemia of 3.8 mmol/L who has been referred to us by A&E.

Background – The patient presented confused and is known to have multiple myeloma. He is under the care of this hospital's oncology services. For the past several days he has been passing large amounts of urine.

Assessment – The patient is responsive to voice and confused. He appeared to be clinically fluid deplete, with a reduced urine output and was tachycardic and hypotensive. He has responded to a fluid challenge and I have commenced him on a rehydration regimen with 0.9 % NaCl running at 250 ml/hour.

Recommendations – I would be grateful if you could come and review this patient. Is there anything you would like me to do in the meantime?

Acute hypercalcaemia in brief

1. What is the pathophysiology of acute hypercalcaemia secondary to malignancy?
Various tumours (particularly lung squamous cell carcinoma) secrete parathyroid hormone-related peptides (PTHrP), which stimulate osteoclasts to resorb bone and suppress osteoblastic bone formation. As a result, excessive calcium is released into the serum from the skeletal stores. In addition, PTHrP reduces the renal excretion of calcium and increases the excretion of phosphate leading to hypophosphataemia.

In the presence of multiple bony metastases or multiple myeloma, the local release of inflammatory mediators such as cytokines (IL-1, IL-6) and PTHrP stimulates osteoclastic bone resorption releasing skeletally stored calcium into the serum, which overwhelms the kidney's excretory capability.

Malignant cells may also over-express 1-alpha hydroxylase leading to overproduction of bioactive vitamin D, which increases intestinal calcium absorption and stimulates osteoclastic bone resorption.

2. What are the common causes of hypercalcaemia?
- Primary and secondary hyperparathyroidism
- Thyrotoxicosis
- Non-blood malignancies (breast, renal, lung squamous cell, ovarian, endometrial)
- Blood malignancies (lymphomas, multiple myeloma)
- Sarcoidosis
- Tuberculosis
- Vitamin D and lithium intoxication

3. How can you differentiate biochemically between hypercalcaemia caused by multiple myeloma and bony metastases?

Multiple myeloma:
- Increased serum adjusted calcium
- Increased or normal serum phosphate
- Normal serum alkaline phosphate

Metastatic disease:
- Increased serum adjusted calcium
- Reduced serum phosphate
- Increase serum alkaline phosphate

Case 4 – **Tumour Lysis Syndrome**

You are a Foundation Year 1 doctor working on the oncology ward. You are asked to see Frances Thomas, a 26 year-old woman, who was recently diagnosed with a highly aggressive non-Hodgkin's lymphoma. Two days ago she was admitted to hospital and started on high intensity chemotherapy. She has now become unwell and is complaining of severe nausea, vomiting and diarrhoea.

Please perform an A to E assessment of Miss Thomas and commence the initial management.

Latest observations:
HR: 120 BP: 120/75 RR: 20 SaO$_2$: 98 % (RA) Temp: 36.5 °C UO: 150 mL dark urine over 8 hr

Danger
It is safe to approach the patient

Response
Miss Thomas is confused but is responsive to voice

Airway
Look – some vomit around the mouth
Feel – no foreign bodies in the mouth
Listen – no added sound
Treat – suction the excess vomit
Reassess – the airway appears clear

Breathing
Look – appears unwell, dyspnoeic, sitting up in bed
Feel – trachea is central; symmetrical chest expansion; resonant to percussion bilaterally
Listen – vesicular breath sounds bilaterally
Measure – RR 20 SaO$_2$ 98 % (RA)
Treat – no treatment necessary at present, monitor for any signs of deterioration

Circulation
Look – dry mucous membranes, looks cachectic and pale with conjunctival pallor.
Feel – regular, low volume pulse, reduced skin turgor.
Listen – heart sounds normal.
Measure – HR 120; BP 120/75; Temp: 37.0 °C, U/O: 150mL of dark urine over 8 hr.
Treat – obtain IV access, commence fluid therapy and adjust according to fluid balance and electrolytes. Insert a urinary catheter.
Reassess – the patient improves haemodynamically: HR 105, BP 130/80; however, she will require more fluids as she is vomiting and is fluid deplete (See Box 1).

Further investigations:
You review Miss Thomas's bloods that were done earlier that day and notice the following abnormalities:
- Serum uric acid – 8.0 (2.4 – 6.0 mg/dL)
- Serum phosphate – 2.0 (0.8 – 1.4 mmol/L)
- Serum potassium – 6.5 (3.5 – 5.3 mmol/L)
- Serum adj. calcium – 1.5 (2.25 – 2.5 mmol/L)
- Serum LDH – 400 (140 – 280 U/L)
- Serum Creatinine – 200 (baseline <80 mmol/L)
- Serum Urea – 15 (2.5 – 7.1 mmol/L)
- ECG - prolongation of the PR interval

From the above clinical and biochemical findings it becomes apparent that this patient has tumour lysis syndrome triggered by the recent chemotherapy and the resulting acute kidney injury. She will require continuous cardiac monitoring, as the biochemical abnormalities put her at risk of cardiac arrhythmias as well as aggressive fluid replacement (see Box 1).

Box 1. **Management of Tumour Lysis Syndrome (TLS)**

It is easier to prevent tumour lysis syndrome than to treat it. Therefore patients should be carefully evaluated and commenced on prophylactic treatment, prior to the initiation of chemotherapy.

Any hyperkalaemia with associated ECG changes should be urgently treated. Please see the chapter on hyperkalaemia for further details. Plenty of intravenous fluids will increase the glomerular filtration rate and reduce the serum potassium, phosphate and uric acid levels. The amount and rate of fluid administration should be guided by the patient's fluid status and urinary output. If despite adequate fluid therapy there is no increase in urine output, loop diuretics such as furosemide may be used. However, they should not be given to fluid deplete patients, as they will lead to further fluid loss.

Allopurinol or rasburicase can be used to lower the serum concentration of uric acid and reduce the risk of urate-associated nephropathy. Phosphate binders such as aluminium salts can be used to reduce the intestinal phosphate absorption. Patients with electrolyte abnormalities resistant to medical management, fluid overload, severe acidosis, uraemia or seizures should be transferred to HDU/ITU and commenced on dialysis.

Disability

AVPU – Patient is responsive to voice/GCS 13 (E3, V4, M6)
Glucose – 9.8 mmol/L
Pupils/neurology – equal and reactive to light, moving all four limbs

Exposure

There are no rashes. There are a number of rubbery, non-tender lymph nodes in the right posterior triangle of the neck. On abdominal examination there is hepatosplenomegaly of 5cm below the costal margin.

Hand over the patient to Dr Jones (Acute oncology SpR)

Situation – Hello, My name is Dr_____and I am the oncology FY1. I am calling regarding Miss Thomas, a 26 year-old woman who I suspect has developed tumour lysis syndrome.

Background – She has recently been diagnosed with an aggressive form of non-Hodgkin's lymphoma and was admitted several days ago to our ward and commenced on high intensity chemotherapy.

Assessment – On examination she appeared unwell and was vomiting. She was also clinically fluid deplete, with a poor urinary output and a regular tachycardia of 120 bpm, but maintaining her blood pressure. This has improved following a fluid challenge. Her morning blood tests showed high potassium, phosphate, LDH and uric acid, with a low calcium and acute kidney injury. Her ECG showed prolongation of the PR interval. She received 10% of calcium gluconate and nebulised salbutamol and she is now on 0.9% saline infusion. I have also commenced her on allopurinol and aluminium salts.

Recommendations – I would like you to come and review this lady as soon as possible, as I think she is very unwell. Is there anything you would like me to do in the meantime?

Tumour lysis syndrome in brief

1. What is tumour lysis syndrome (TLS)?
Tumour lysis syndrome is an umbrella term for a range of biochemical abnormalities, which are almost exclusively seen in cancer patients, commonly after the initiation of cytotoxic chemotherapy. The chemotherapy causes extensive cell destruction leading to hyperkalaemia, hyperphosphataemia, hyperuricaemia and hypocalcaemia. It is an oncological emergency since the metabolic and electrolyte derangements can lead to cardiac arrhythmias, seizures, lactic acidosis and acute kidney injury.

2. What are the common causes of tumour lysis syndrome?
Tumour lysis syndrome occurs most frequently in haematological malignancies, particularly non-Hodgkin's lymphoma and acute myeloid and lymphocytic leukaemias. This is because these malignancies are characterised by a high cell proliferation rate. However, it can occur with solid tumours, such as breast, lung and testicular cancers, but this is much less common.

3. What is the pathophysiology of tumour lysis syndrome?

Tumour lysis syndrome is more likely to occur in patients with malignancies that show high cell turnover, high tumour bulk and a good response to chemotherapy. In TLS the rapid destruction of cancer cells by cytotoxic agents leads to the release of intracellular content into the blood, which results in the characteristic biochemical abnormalities. Moreover, rapidly dividing malignant cells produce more byproducts of nucleic acid metabolism, which are eventually metabolised into uric acid and phosphate.

Hyperuricaemia and hyperphosphataemia lead to precipitation of uric acid and calcium phosphate crystals respectively in the renal tubules, which may eventually lead to renal obstruction and acute kidney injury. Hypocalcaemia occurs in secondary hyperphosphataemia and if severe can lead to muscle cramps, tetany and seizures. Hyperkalaemia puts the patients at risk of cardiac arrhythmias and sudden death, and should be treated as a matter of urgency. Eventually, acute kidney injury can lead to lactic acidosis, fluid overload, heart failure and pulmonary oedema.

Haematological Emergencies

Sana Owais Subhan

Transfusion Reactions	212
Sickle Cell Crisis	218

Case 1 – **Transfusion Reactions**

You are a Foundation Year 1 doctor on a busy care of the elderly ward. One of the nurses asks you to review, Mrs Amersham, a 75 year old lady. She says Mrs Amersham is feeling very unwell and complaining of chills and pain in her left arm. You saw Mrs Amersham earlier on the ward round. She had a total hip replacement yesterday. Your consultant asked for a transfusion as her haemoglobin level was low. It was started 30 minutes ago. She has a history of osteoarthritis and gastro-oesophageal reflux disease and has no known allergies.

Please conduct an A to E assessment of Mrs Amersham and commence the initial management.

Latest observations:
HR 106, BP 117/72, RR 20, SaO_2 99 % (RA), Temp 38.1 °C, UO: 650 mL (8 hours)

Danger
It is safe to approach the patient

Response
The patient responds: "Doctor, I feel very cold."

Airway
The airway is patent

Breathing
Look – no use of accessory muscles
Feel – central trachea, normal chest expansion and percussion
Listen – vesicular breath sounds and bilateral equal air entry
Measure – RR 20 SaO_2 99 % (RA)
Treat – no need for treatment

Circulation
Look – shivering, flushed, sweaty
Feel – CRT <3 seconds
Listen – normal heart sounds
Measure – HR 106, BP 117/72, Temp 38.1°C, U/O 650 mL
Treat – stop the transfusion. Give paracetamol for the fever. Restart the infusion of a new sample at a slower rate once the fever has subsided.
Reassess – HR 87, BP 118/70, Temp 37.0, U/O 700 mL

Further investigations:
- Recheck drug chart and blood products to ensure ABO compatibility
- Direct anti-globulin test and post-transfusion urinalysis
- Bloods (FBC, U&E, clotting D-Dimer and fibrinogen) and resend 2 crossmatch samples

Disability
AVPU – alert/ GCS 15 (E4V5M6)
Check glucose – 4.9 mmol/L
Pupils – equal and reactive

Exposure
There is a widespread erythematous rash but nothing else of note is seen.
The abdomen is soft and non-tender. Consider giving the patient an antihistamine such as chlorphenomine for the rash.

Hand over patient to Dr Tanaka (Haematology SpR)

Situation – Hello Dr Tanaka, this is _____, the FY1 in care of the elderly. I am calling you regarding Mrs Amersham, a 75 year old lady, who has had a febrile non-haemolytic transfusion reaction.

Background – Mrs Amersham had a total hip replacement yesterday. A blood transfusion was started approximately 30 minutes ago as her haemoglobin levels were low. She has a history of osteoarthritis and GORD. She has no known allergies.

Assessment – On examination, I noted that Mrs Amersham was febrile, with a temperature of 38.1°C, and tachycardic at 106 bpm. I stopped the transfusion and started her on IV paracetamol. Her temperature and her heart rate have gone down.

I have also looked over the drug chart and rechecked the patient's ABO compatibility, and found no discrepancies. I have sent off a direct anti-globulin test, FBC and U&E. I have also done a urinalysis, which showed no haemoglobinuria.

Recommendation – I would appreciate it if you could come and review Mrs Amersham. I intend to start a different unit of blood at a slower rate once she is afebrile. In the meantime, is there anything else you would like me to do?

Transfusion reactions in brief

1. What are the different types of transfusion reactions and how can they be managed?

IMMUNE MEDIATED – ACUTE (<24 HOURS)

a) Acute haemolytic transfusion reaction

Usually presents within 15 minutes of the start of the transfusion. It is characterised by fever, chills, rigors and haemoglobinuria. Patients may experience pain along the site of access or chest and abdomen. It can be associated with tachycardia, hypotension, renal failure and disseminated intravascular coagulopathy (DIC). The severity of the reaction depends on how long the patient has been transfused for and the amount of blood volume received.

Management: Stop the transfusion → fluid resuscitate with normal saline (aim for urine output >100 ml/hr)

b) Allergic reaction

Presents within minutes of starting the transfusion, with urticaria, flushing and a rash. Sometimes angioedema can develop.

Management: temporarily stop the blood transfusion → give antihistamines. If reaction is severe: give corticosteroids and closely monitor for onset of anaphylaxis. Discuss the patient with your seniors. Transfusion should not be restarted.

c) Anaphylactic reaction

The onset is usually within the first hour of the transfusion. Patients may have: nausea, vomiting, hypotension and respiratory distress, amongst other signs.

Management: Stop the transfusion → give IM adrenaline +/- airway support +/- inhaled bronchodilator +/- anti histamine +/- corticosteroids.

d) Febrile non-haemolytic transfusion reaction

Patients present with a fever, and at least a 1 °C rise from the pre-transfusion temperature. They may also experience nausea, headaches and chills, but are generally quite well.

Management: Stop the transfusion temporarily → give antipyretics → Restart a new blood unit after any other reaction has been ruled out. Do not re-transfuse remainder of previous one.

e) Transfusion-related acute lung injury

Usually occurs within 1 to 2 hours after the transfusion, but can manifest itself up to 6 hours after. An autoimmune reaction causes an increase in pulmonary vasculature permeability leading to pulmonary oedema, tachypnoea and dyspnoea as well as fever and tachycardia.

Management: Stop the transfusion → supportive care (can range from oxygen therapy to mechanical ventilation, depending on the severity). Usually resolves within 7 days.

IMMUNE MEDIATED - DELAYED (>24 HOURS)

a) Delayed haemolytic transfusion reaction

The symptoms may develop days to weeks after transfusion. Patient presents with jaundice, fever, low haemoglobin and fatigue. A urine dipstick may demonstrate haemoglobinuria.

Management: Supportive care → fluid resuscitate with normal saline (urine output >100ml/hr)

b) Transfusion associated graft-versus-host disease

The onset is usually 7 – 10 days after the transfusion. Classically associated with a maculopapular rash. Patients may also experience fever and diarrhoea. Unfortunately, the prognosis is poor.

Management: supportive care with immunosuppressive therapy and prior irradiation of transfusion products.

c) Post transfusion purpura

Usually occurs during pregnancy, leading to a widespread purpura and bleeding from mucous membranes. Occurs 8 – 10 days after transfusion.

Management: Intravenous immunoglobulins

NON-IMMUNE MEDIATED

a) Transfusion associated sepsis

Usually occurs within 4 hours of the transfusion and results from bacterial contamination of blood products. Patients may experience fever, nausea and vomiting. They may also present with septic shock or disseminated intravascular coagulopathy.

Management: Stop the transfusion → symptomatic treatment → blood cultures and antibiotics

b) Transfusion associated circulatory overload

Occurs within hours of the transfusion. Patients may experience breathing difficulties like orthopnoea, cough productive of pink frothy sputum, headache and hypertension.

Management: Stop the transfusion → sit the patient up → oxygen therapy → diuretics (monitor fluid balance). Perform a chest x-ray.

Case 2 – **Sickle Cell Crisis**

You are a Foundation Year 2 doctor working in the Emergency Department. You have been asked to see a 27 year old man, Jensen Worthington, with known sickle cell disease. He is complaining of severe right sided hip pain which started two hours ago. He has also vomited 3 times. He tried to manage it with ibuprofen but says it did not touch the pain. He has no other history of note or any drug allergies.

Please conduct an A to E assessment of Jensen Worthington and commence the initial management.

Latest observations:

HR 77, BP 100/65, RR 22, SaO_2 95 % (RA), Temp 36.4 °C, UO: NA

Danger

It is safe to approach the patient.

Response

The patient is alert and talking to you.

Airway

The patient is talking so you can assume the airway is patent.

Breathing

Look – no use of accessory muscles
Feel – central trachea, normal chest expansion and percussion
Listen – vesicular breath sounds and bilateral equal air entry
Measure – RR 22, SaO$_2$ 95 % (on room air)
Treat – monitor for oxygen desaturation. Move on.

Circulation

Look – flushed, sweaty
Feel – CRT <3 seconds, warm to touch
Listen – normal heart sounds
Measure – HR 77, BP 100/65, temp 36.4 °C, U/O: not available
Treat – obtain IV access and rehydrate the patient with fluids. Give strong analgesia (e.g. morphine)
Reassess – pain has settled slightly

Disability

AVPU – alert/ GCS15 (E4V5M6)
Blood glucose – 5.3 mmol/L
Pupils – equal and reactive to light

Exposure

The right hip is very tender with reduced range of both active and passive motion.

Hand over patient to Dr Corben (Haematology SpR)

Situation – Hello Dr Corben, this is _____, the FY2 in A&E. I am calling you regarding Jensen Worthington, a 27 year old man, with known sickle cell disease who I believe presents with a vaso-occlusive sickle cell crisis.

Background – Mr Worthington presented with a two-hour severe right-sided hip pain and 3 episodes of vomiting. He took some ibuprofen which did not alleviate the pain. He has no other associated symptoms.

Assessment – On examination, Mr Worthington appeared unwell with a heart rate of 77 and a blood pressure of 100/65. He was mildly tachypnoeic, with a respiratory rate of 22, and saturations of 95 % on room air. I obtained IV access and started him on morphine for his pain and rehydration with crystalloid fluids.

Recommendation – I would appreciate it if you could come and review Mr Worthington. In the meantime, is there anything else you would like me to do?

Sickle cell anaemia in brief

1. What is sickle cell anaemia?

An autosomal recessive disease of the red blood cells, which is caused by a gene mutation in the beta chain of haemoglobin A (HbA), with the valine replacing glutamic acid at the 6th amino acid position. This leads to formation of haemoglobin S (HbS). It is more common in the Afro-Caribbean population as it confers protection against malaria in endemic regions. The abnormal red cells change shape in hypoxic and acidotic conditions into crescent-shaped cells (ie. sickle cells). This leads to anaemia and disruption of blood flow as a result of microvascular occlusion by the sickle cells. This results in a sickle cell crisis, with patients presenting with severe pain and end-organ damage.

2. What are the common complications of sickle cell anaemia and how should they be managed?

- **Pulmonary hypertension** – treated with calcium channel blockers (nifedipine or diltiazem), endothelin receptor antagonists (bosentan), phosphodiesterase-5 inhibitors (sildenafil) and prostacyclin infusion.
- **Splenic sequestration** – treated with red blood cell transfusions and splenectomy
- **Splenic infarction** – requires pneumococcal, haemophilus, meningococcal and influenza vaccines
- **Cholelithiasis** – treated with elective cholecystectomy
- **Avascular necrosis of the femoral head** – treated with pain relief and arthroplasty
- **Dactylitis** – requires good hydration and analgesia
- **Priapism** – if an episode lasts longer than 4 hours it is considered an urological emergency and should be treated with analgesia, injections with sympathomimetic agents, aspiration or surgical decompression.
- **Iron overload** – treated with iron sequestration agents (deferoxamine)
- **Leg ulceration** – treated with hydration, elevation and zinc sulphate pressure dressings

Poisoning Emergencies

Ersong Shang

Benzodiazepines and Tricyclic Antidepressants Overdose	224
Cardiovascular Drug Overdose	230
Opioid Overdose	234
Stimulant Overdose	238
Carbon Monoxide and Cyanide Poisoning	244

Case 1 – **Benzodiazepines and Tricyclic Antidepressants Overdose**

You are a Foundation Year 2 doctor working in A&E. A 23 year old Laura Miller is found collapsed at home after breaking up with her boyfriend and is brought in by ambulance. She has a history of depression with previous self-harm episodes and a personality disorder. A suicide note is found next to her with several empty medication boxes and a bottle of vodka. The ambulance crew has started the patient on high flow oxygen via a non-rebreathe mask as she was desaturating on room air. They hand you over the empty medication boxes, which suggests that she has taken a lot of diazepam and amitriptyline.

Please conduct an A to E assessment of Ms Miller and commence the initial management.

Latest observations:
HR:110, BP:110/85, RR:10, SaO_2: 99 % (15 L of O_2), temp: 37.3 °C, UO: NA

Danger

Safe to approach patient.

Response

The patient responds to pain, it is appropriate to call for help at this stage.

Airway

Look – no foreign objects or vomit in the mouth, oxygen mask is fogging up
Feel – nil
Listen – patient is snoring
Treat – no suspicion of cervical spine injury, perform a head-tilt-chin-lift
Reassess – patient is no longer snoring, and maintaining her own airway

Breathing

Look – no cyanosis
Feel – chest is resonant to percussion and expansion is symmetrical bilaterally
Listen – normal vesicular breath sounds throughout both lung fields
Measure – RR 10, SaO_2 99 % on 15 L O_2 via non-rebreathe mask
Treat – reduce O_2 therapy, aiming for SaO_2 94-98%
Reassess – patient is stable, move on

Further investigations

- Perform an ABG - shows a raised anion gap metabolic acidosis

Circulation

Look – appears to be flushed and dry, there is no pallor or clamminess
Feel – the patient feels hot to touch, CRT <2 seconds
Listen – heart sounds I and II are heard with no added sounds
Measure – HR 80 regular, BP 110/85
Treat – obtain intravenous access and consider starting an IV HCO_3^- infusion to correct the acidosis following a discussion with your senior
Reassess – HCO_3^- infusion is commenced, patient is no longer hypoxic and not hypotensive. Ensure the patient is placed on a cardiac-monitored bed to check for dynamic ECG changes. Regular blood gas analysis should be used to guide HCO_3^- therapy, aiming for a pH of 7.5 – 7.55

Further investigations:
- ECG – prolongation of the PR interval, broadening of the QRS complex, corrected QT interval is 480 ms.

The ECG changes and metabolic acidosis are in keeping with severe overdose with tricyclic antidepressants. Even though the patient maybe haemodynamically stable for now, she is at risk of developing life threatening arrhythmias. To reduce this risk one should treat her hypoxia, fluid resuscitate the patient and consider correcting the acidosis with IV HCO_3^- infusion following a discussion with your seniors.

Disability

AVPU – patient is responsive to pain/GCS 9 (E2V3M4)
Capillary blood glucose – 7 mmol/L
Pupils/neurology – dilated, poorly reactive to light. There is hypertonia and hyperreflexia in all 4 limbs, with bilaterally upgoing plantars and ankle clonus but no evidence of focal neurology.

Exposure

No other injuries or evidence of deliberate self-harm were found.

A dull mass arising out of the pelvis was palpated in the abdomen. This was confirmed as an enlarged bladder and the patient was catheterised, draining 600mL of clear urine.

Further investigations:
- Blood and urine toxicology screen

Refer to Toxbase® for further information on various poisons and substances (https://www.toxbase.org). Your hospital should have the access details

A psychiatric risk assessment should then be performed assessing further risk of self-harming behaviour and the patient should be referred to the local liaison psychiatry team.

Hand over the patient to Dr Shang (Critical Care SpR)

Situation – Hello Dr Shang, this is Dr _____, an FY2 in A&E. I have just seen a 23 year old Laura Miller, brought in by ambulance with a GCS of 9 after a suspected mixed overdose of amitriptyline and diazepam with vodka.

Background – She is thought to have taken an intentional overdose. The time of the overdose is unknown. She was commenced on 15 L of oxygen via a non-rebreathe mask in the ambulance as her initial SaO_2 was 90 % on air. She has a past history of depression with episodes of self-harm and a personality disorder.

Assessment – Her initial observations were HR: 110, BP 110/85, RR 10, SaO_2 is 99 % on 15 L, temp 37.3 °C. Heart sounds were normal however, an ECG demonstrated prolonged PR, QRS and QT intervals. An arterial blood gas showed a high anion gap metabolic acidosis. She was in urinary retention and was catheterised. Her pupils are dilated, and she has generalised hypertonia and hyper-reflexia, bilaterally up going plantars and ankle clonus. We have continued oxygen therapy and she is maintaining her airway. Her capillary blood glucose is 7.

Recommendation – I believe this patient is highly unstable and needs critical care input for continued monitoring and stabilisation. Would you please come and assess this patient as soon as possible.

Benzodiazepines and tricyclic antidepressants overdose in brief

1. Why are benzodiazepines dangerous in overdose, and what is the management?

Benzodiazepine overdose suppresses the patients' respiratory drive and leads to a compromised airway. Therefore these patients may require intubation and respiratory support. Flumazenil can be used to reverse the effects of benzodiazepine overdose. However, in practice it is rarely used, as reversing the effects of benzodiazepine lowers the patient's seizure threshold, putting them at risk of seizures. Furthermore, in a mixed overdose with anticholinergic drugs patients are predisposed to seizures.

2. What other drugs can patients with depression overdose on, and how are they managed?

Barbiturate overdose is managed with similar supportive measures to benzodiazepine overdose. However the use of barbiturates has declined because of the narrow therapeutic range of these drugs as well as multiple drug interactions and side effects. Following an overdose, barbiturates can be removed by haemodialysis if necessary. Agents that can be removed by haemodialysis are recalled by the acronym "BLAST": barbiturates, lithium, alcohols, salicylates and theophylline.

3. What is an anticholinergic toxidrome?

This patient presented classically with the anticholinergic toxidrome caused by tricyclic antidepressants, the symptoms of which include: dry mouth, urinary retention (both are early signs), decreased level of consciousness, fever, increased tone, hyper-reflexia, and clonus. Anticholinergic toxicity can also predispose to seizure activity, so flumazenil must not be given.

4. What are the most serious complications of anticholinergic toxicity?

It is the cardiovascular effects of anticholinergics that are of great concern and should be managed as a priority. Patients can become tachycardic and hypotensive, with the ECG demonstrating prolongation of the PR interval, broadening of the QRS complexes and prolongation of the corrected QT interval. These electrical changes within the conduction system of the heart will predispose the patient to fatal arrhythmias and can cause a cardiac arrest. This can be prevented by correcting any pre-existing hypoxia and hypotension and in cases of metabolic acidosis or ECG changes an 8.4 % HCO_3^- infusion must be started with the aim to maintain the arterial pH between 7.5 – 7.55.

5. What is the role of gastric lavage in tricyclic antidepressant overdose?

Anticholinergic overdose is one of the few occasions where gastric lavage may be used 1 hour post ingestion due to its gastro-static anticholinergic effects. However gastric lavage must be carried out under senior supervision following appropriate training and with correct equipment.

Case 2 – **Cardiovascular Drug Overdose**

You are a Foundation Year 2 doctor working in A&E. A 73-year-old Beth Wilson is brought in by ambulance after being found unconscious. She has a known history of depression and anxiety, as well as fast atrial fibrillation, which is being rate-controlled by her GP. According to the ambulance crew she is suspected to have taken an intentional overdose of propranolol. The quantity and timing of the overdose cannot be confirmed at this point. No other past medical history is available.

Please conduct an A to E assessment of Mrs Wilson and commence the initial management.

Latest observations:

HR: 35 BP: 80/45 RR: 22 SaO$_2$: 92 % (RA) Temp: 36.5 °C U/O: NA

Danger

It is safe to approach the patient

Response

The patient is responsive to pain. Ask for assistance at this point.

Airway

Look – no visible obstructions or vomitus
Feel – trachea is central
Listen – patient is snoring
Treat – no cervical spine injury is suspected, therefore perform a head-tilt-chin-lift manoeuvre. If this fails use an oropharyngeal or nasopharyngeal airway.
Reassess – the patient is no longer snoring and seems able to tolerate the oropharyngeal airway. Carefully monitor her airway.

Breathing

Look – chest is moving symmetrically, peripheral cyanosis is noted
Feel – breaths are felt, equal chest expansion, resonant percussion
Listen – bilateral wheeze and bibasal crepitations
Measure – RR 22, SaO_2 92 % on air
Treat – 5 mg nebulised salbutamol, driven by oxygen
Reassess – RR 16, SaO_2 98 % Perform regular chest auscultations to monitor if the wheeze subsides with salbutamol therapy.

Further investigations:
- Perform an ABG – mild lactic acidosis

Circulation

Look – patient looks pale
Feel – cold to touch, bradycardic, low volume pulse, pitting oedema up to mid shin
Listen – normal heart sounds
Measure – HR 35, BP 80/45, temp 36.5 °C, CRT 5s, UO: NA
Treat – obtain IV access, administer a fluid challenge with NaCl 0.9 %, 500 ml over 15 minutes (up to 2000 ml). Consider IV atropine or glucagon to increase HR.
Reassess – HR 60, BP 100/60, continue monitoring the ECG and blood pressure; reassess the patient's fluid status and consider further fluids.

Further investigations:
- ECG – sinus bradycardia, no evidence of ischaemia
- Bloods (FBC, U&E, LFTs, troponin)
- Place the patient on a cardiac monitor

If atropine fails to increase the heart rate, glucagon should be tried. Other forms of ionotropic/chronotropic support may be used and temporary pacing may be needed in resistant cases.

Disability

AVPU – patient responsive to pain/ GCS 8 (E2V2M4)
Capillary blood glucose – 7 mmol/L
Pupils – equal and reactive to light, tone and reflexes are normal bilaterally

Even though the patient is currently maintaining their airway with an oropharyngeal airway adjunct, intubation may be required with a GCS of 8. An anaesthetist should therefore be called.

Exposure

Abdomen is soft and non-tender, bowel sounds present. There are no indications of trauma, no evidence of deliberate self-harm.

Further investigations:
- Blood and urine toxicology screen

Refer to Toxbase® for further information on various poisons and substances (https://www.toxbase.org). Your hospital should have the access details.

Hand over the patient to Dr Wilkins (Medical SpR):

Situation – Hello Dr Wilkins, this is Dr_____ the FY2 working in A&E. I have just seen a 73-year-old Beth Wilson who has been brought in by ambulance having been found unconscious secondary to a suspected intentional beta-blocker overdose, which resulted in a cardiogenic shock.

Background – she was found by her neighbours unconscious with some empty propranolol boxes. The time and amount of overdose are unknown. She has a past history of anxiety and depression and fast AF which is being rate-controlled by her GP. Other past medical history is unclear at this point.

Assessment – On initial assessment she was only responsive to pain with a GCS of 8 (E2V2M4). She was maintaining her airway with an oropharyngeal airway. Her ECG showed sinus bradycardia with an HR of 35 and no evidence of ischaemia. She has a mild wheeze bilaterally that improved following 5mg of nebulised salbutamol therapy. The patient had a capillary blood glucose of 7 mmol and no focal neurology. So far we have given this patient 500 mL of fluids IV, atropine and glucagon IV. We have sent off bloods, as well as a blood and urine toxicology screen, and her ABG showed mild lactic acidosis.

Recommendation – The patient has responded very well to atropine and glucagon and is now alert and cardiovascularly stable. However I would like for her to be admitted under the medical team for further monitoring.

Cardiovascular drug overdose in brief

1. What are the features of a beta-blocker overdose and how is it managed?
Beta-blockers generally cause a sinus bradycardia and in severe cases will lead to cardiogenic shock and heart failure (as in this patient). The treatment is with intravenous glucagon, which is a good antidote. The presentation will vary depending on the type of beta-blocker consumed. An overdose with a non-selective beta-blocker such as propranolol will cause bronchospasm, which can be treated with nebulised salbutamol. Sotalol, whilst a beta blocker, is classified as a type III anti-arrhythmic in the Vaughan Williams classification, and as such it will cause prolongation of the QRS and QT intervals, that could lead to torsade de pointes and ventricular tachycardia.

2. What are the features of a calcium-channel blocker overdose and how is it managed?
Overdose with calcium channel blockers is considered more serious since treatment is more challenging. The dihydropyridine class, which includes amlodipine, will cause cardiovascular collapse by vasodilation. On the other hand, the non-dihydropyridine class will lead to cardiovascular collapse by blocking the AV node and reducing cardiac output. However, at very high doses the class-specific actions of these drugs are lost and the effects are a combination of peripheral vasodilation with AV-nodal block. Atropine is the mainstay of treatment but glucagon may also be effective in certain cases. In a severe overdose, IV calcium infusion, ionotropic support and pacing may be needed. It must be noted that a calcium infusion can only be given if digoxin toxicity has been ruled out.

3. What are the features of digoxin toxicity and how is it managed?
Digoxin toxicity is rare but extremely dangerous. In elderly patients it may occur due to a medication error, reduced renal function or electrolyte imbalance. In children it may be due to accidental consumption of cardiac glycoside-containing plants. Digoxin toxicity leads to nausea, vomiting, delirium and xanthopsia. ECG changes consistent with digoxin toxicity include bradycardia, AV nodal block, AV dissociation, ventricular ectopics, prolongation of QRS complex and ventricular tachycardia. It is important to note that the "reverse tick" ST segment depression indicates the use of digoxin but not overdose. Sometimes digoxin overdose may be treated with a digoxin specific antibody, however expert opinion should be sought regarding its necessity and use.

Case 3 – **Opioid Overdose**

You are a Foundation Year 2 doctor working in A&E. You are asked to urgently see a 28-year-old patient, Sam Smith, who is brought in by the ambulance. Mr Smith was found unconscious on the street with a set of syringes next to him. He is well known to the ambulance crews and triage nurses from past admissions and is a known intra-venous drug user.

Please conduct an A to E assessment of Mr Smith and commence the initial management.

Latest observations:
HR: 105, BP: 100/60, RR: 8, SaO_2: 92 % (on room air), temp: 36.5 °C, UO: NA

Danger

It is safe to approach Mr Smith. However, you notice that the patient appears unkempt and there are multiple needle-track marks on his arms and legs. You should therefore wear gloves and take extra care to avoid exposure to patient's bodily fluids and blood-borne viruses.

Response

Patient groans to pain, it is appropriate to call for help as this stage.

Airway

Look – no visible obstruction or loose objects in the mouth
Feel – trachea central, breaths are felt
Listen – faint breath sounds are heard and the patient is snoring
Treat – perform a head-tilt chin-lift manoeuvre and consider an oropharyngeal or a nasopharyngeal airway.
Reassess – the patient is now maintaining his airway

Breathing

Look – chest is moving, patient appears centrally cyanosed
Feel – chest is resonant to percussion, but with reduced symmetrical expansion
Listen – vesicular breath sounds are heard bilaterally with no added sounds
Measure – RR: 8, SaO_2: 92 % (on room air)
Treat – since patient is unconscious with RR <10, he should be ventilated with a bag-valve mask at 10 – 12 breaths per minute connected to high flow O_2
Reassess – breath sounds are heard bilaterally, SaO_2 has improved to 100 % on 15 L via bag valve mask, patient is no longer cyanosed

Further investigations:
- Perform an ABG – respiratory acidosis

Circulation

Look – no pallor, nor clamminess
Feel – patient feels slightly cool peripherally and sweaty
Listen – normal heart sounds
Measure – BP 100/60, weak but regular pulse at 105, CRT <2 seconds
Treat – obtain IV access, fluid resuscitate with a crystalloid.
Reassess – BP is responsive to fluid resuscitation and HR decrease. Administer further fluid resuscitation.

Further investigations:
- ECG – sinus rhythm with no acute changes

Disability

AVPU – patient is responsive to pain/GCS 8 (E2V2M4)
Capillary blood glucose – 7 mmol/L
Pupils – pin point and not responsive to light, there appears to be no focal neurology

A diagnosis of opioid overdose should be considered, and naloxone must be titrated according to response. Initially 400 micrograms is given intravenously. This may have to be repeated every 3 min up to 10 mg as naloxone has a short half-life of approximately 60 min.

The patient regains full consciousness over the next 5 minutes and RR goes up to 20. SaO_2 100 % on high flow oxygen (consider reducing the O_2 flow rate).

Exposure

On full exposure you note multiple needle-track marks on upper and lower limbs. There are several ulcers on the lower limbs. No other injuries are noted, and the abdomen is soft and non-tender with bowel sounds present. No head injury is noted.

Further investigations:
- Blood and urine toxicology screen

Refer to Toxbase® for further information on various poisons and substances (https://www.toxbase.org). Your hospital should have the access details.

Hand over the patient to Dr Kannani (A&E SpR)

Situation – My name is Dr_____ and I am the FY2 in A&E. I would like to discuss Mr Sam Smith, a 28-year-old patient who has taken an opioid overdose.

Background – The patient was brought in by ambulance after being found unconscious on the street with some syringes next to him. He is well-known to the ambulance crews and the triage nurses and is a known IVDU.

Assessment – His initial observations were HR: 105, BP: 100/60, RR: 8, SaO$_2$: 92 % (on room air), temp: 36.5 °C. He had normal heart sounds. His respiratory effort was weak, but air entry was equal bilaterally. The abdomen was soft and non-tender. He had pinpoint pupils, which were unreactive to light. There was no focal neurology of note. Based on my assessment I diagnosed opioid overdose and proceeded to bag and valve mask ventilation, and have given naloxone IV to help reverse the opioid overdose. He responded to treatment and has regained consciousness. His most recent observations are HR: 80, BP: 115/70, RR: 20, SaO$_2$: 100 % (on 15 L O$_2$), temp: 36.5 °C, UO: not available, capillary blood glucose: 7 mmol/L.

Recommendations – I would like you to review this patient. In the meantime I was planning on continuing the oxygen and naloxone therapy. Is there anything else you would like me to do?

Opioid overdose in brief

1. What predisposes patients to opioid overdose?

Opioid overdose is common in patients who misuse illicit drugs such as heroin or methadone. However, therapeutic overdose can also occur in a hospital setting. Elderly, underweight and opioid naïve patients are especially susceptible. In such patients doctors should consider starting the drug at a lower dose (e.g. 2.5 – 5 mg of morphine sulphate oral solution) and titrate upwards according to patient's response.

Patients with impaired renal function are also susceptible to opioid overdose because of the accumulation of the drug and its metabolically active metabolites. Care must therefore be taken when prescribing both short and long acting opioids in patients with chronic kidney disease or patients at risk of acute kidney injury. Fentanyl and other related opioids are not cleared renally, and are generally considered safe in renal impairment.

2. What is naloxone and what do you have to be aware of when using it?

Naloxone is the drug of choice for the reversal of opioid toxicity, as it is a competitive antagonist at the opioid μ- receptors in the central nervous system. It is generally given intravenously for rapid effect. However, intramuscular naloxone can be used when a longer action is needed or intravenous access cannot be established. Intranasal naloxone is also available and can also be given when intravenous access is not available. It is important to know that naloxone may precipitate a withdrawal-like reaction in opioid dependent patients, leading to agitation and aggression. Naloxone will also reverse the analgesic effects of opioids and therefore opioid overdoses should not be fully reversed in patients who are likely to be in severe pain. Naloxone has a short in vivo half-life when compared to most opioid drugs. As a result patients must not be discharged straight away because the effects of naloxone are likely to wear off post-discharge and patients might relapse into an opioid toxicity state again.

Case 4 – **Stimulant Overdose**

You are a Foundation Year 2 doctor working nights in the Emergency Department. An ambulance has just brought in a 27-year-old Farquhar Johnson after he collapsed and fitted at a night club. According to the ambulance crew he had taken copious amounts of cocaine and MDMA with plenty of alcohol. He is reported to have seized for 3 minutes before the ambulance arrived. He had 2 further episodes whilst in the ambulance each lasting between 3 to 4 minutes, without fully regaining consciousness in between.

Please conduct an A to E assessment of Mr Johnson and commence the initial management.

Latest observations:
HR: 140, BP: 160/90, RR:25, SaO_2: 98 % (on 15 L), temp: 40.1 °C , UO: NA

Danger

Safe to approach the patient

Response

The patient responds to pain, it is appropriate to call for help at this stage

Airway

Look – no visible obstructions or vomit, some blood is noted in the mouth
Feel – trachea is central
Listen – patient is snoring
Treat – Yankauer sucker is used to clear the blood from the mouth, head-tilt-chin-lift is used to open the airway, as there is no suspected cervical spine injury and an oropharyngeal/nasopharyngeal airway is used to maintain the airway
Reassess – patient is no longer snoring, move on

Breathing

Look – no cyanosis, oxygen mask is fogging up as appropriate
Feel – normal chest expansion, resonant percussion
Listen – normal vesicular breaths are heard throughout
Measure – RR 20, SaO_2 98 % on high flow oxygen via a non-rebreathe mask
Treat – reduce O_2 delivery aiming at SaO_2 94-98%

Further investigations:
- Perform an ABG – shows lactic acidosis, slightly elevated K^+.

Circulation

Look – patient does not appear pale or clammy
Feel – patient is warm to touch, CRT <2 seconds
Listen – normal heart sounds
Measure – HR 140, BP160/90, temp 40.1 °C
Treat – obtain IV access, insert a urinary catheter to monitor fluid balance. Cool the patient externally with cool packs around the neck, axilla and groin. Start IV fluid resuscitation to rehydrate the patient, prevent rhabdomyolysis and increase urine output.
Reassess – patient is cardiovascularly stable but will require continuous cardiac monitoring with a 3-lead ECG and frequent blood pressure measurements

Further investigations:
- ECG – sinus tachycardia with no acute changes indicative of ischaemia or an arrhythmia
- Bloods (FBC, U&E, CRP, LFTs, glucose, creatinine, creatinine kinase)
- Blood cultures

Disability

AVPU – patient is responsive to pain/GCS 9 (E2V3M4)
Capillary blood glucose – 8 mmol/L
Pupils/neurology – dilated, poorly reactive to light, mild hypertonia in all 4 limbs with hyper-reflexia and up-going plantars bilaterally

---

If this patient continues to have seizures without regaining full consciousness between episodes, this should be treated as status epilepticus and IV lorazepam should be given. If this fails to terminate the seizures, status epilepticus treatment should be repeated and then escalated (IV lorazepam → IV phenytoin → IV thiopental or propafol). The patient's respiratory function should be carefully monitored because benzodiazepines can cause respiratory depression.

Temperature needs to be monitored and cooling treatment may need to be escalated if temperature continues to rise. IV fluids need to be titrated according to urine output to preserve renal function and lower potassium whilst avoiding pulmonary oedema. Regularly monitor U&Es.

Exposure

There appears to be no signs of injuries. The patient's abdomen is soft and non-tender with bowel sounds present.

Further investigations:
- Blood and urine toxicology screen

Refer to Toxbase® for further information on various poisons and substances (https://www.toxbase.org). Your hospital should have the access details.

Hand over the patient to Dr Shang (Critical Care SpR)

Situation – Hello, this is Dr_____, the FY2 in A&E. I am calling regarding a 27-year-old Farquhar Johnson who has been brought in by ambulance. I suspect he has overdosed on some stimulants.

Background – He is reported to have had 3 witnessed seizure episodes following taking cocaine, MDMA and alcohol at a night club. His friends witnessed one episode and the ambulance crew witnessed two further episodes. Each episode lasted between 3 to 4 minutes and he has not fully regained consciousness in between. He is reported to have taken large amounts of the drugs mentioned above for recreational purposes. There is no evidence of deliberate overdose. The past medical history is as yet unknown.

Assessment – His most recent observations are HR: 140, BP: 160/90, RR: 24, SaO_2: 98 % (on 15 L O_2), temp 40.1 °C, GCS 9. He was snoring and we therefore inserted an oropharyngeal airway which he tolerated. His respiratory assessment was normal, however an ABG had shown a mild lactic acidosis and a K^+ of 5.3 mmol/L. He was tachycardic and his ECG demonstrated sinus tachycardia with no evidence of ischaemia. His pupils are dilated and unresponsive to light. There is increased tone in all 4 limbs with hyper-reflexia and up-going plantars bilaterally.

So far I have started fluid resuscitation to increase his urine output. I have tried to cool him externally with cool packs, however his temperature is still high. He has not seized since admission. I have sent off bloods for FBC, U&E, LFT, clotting, blood glucose, creatinine, creatinine kinase, blood and urine toxicology screen.

Recommendation – I believe this person is exhibiting evidence of serotonin syndrome as a result of his overdose. I would like for you to come and assess this patient for escalation of treatment and admission to ITU as soon as possible.

Stimulant overdose in brief

1. Give some examples of stimulant recreational drugs
- Amphetamine
- Methamphetamine
- MDMA (Ecstasy)
- Cocaine
- Caffeine
- Nicotine

2. What are the common effects of stimulant drugs?
Whilst the types of stimulants being used and abused are always changing as new 'legal highs' are discovered and older stimulants go out of fashion, the basic effects are very similar. They all activate the adrenergic system to produce feelings of euphoria, loss of inhibition, boundless energy, confidence, sometimes aggression or excessive friendliness.

3. What are the features of MDMA toxicity and how is it managed?
MDMA (3,4-methylenedioxymethamphetamine) also commonly known as ecstasy is an amphetamine derivative. In overdose it has an effect on multiple systems including the central nervous, cardiovascular and gastrointestinal systems. Toxicity leads to restlessness, anxiety, change in mental status, headache, ataxia, blurred vision and seizures. Patients may experience abdominal pain with nausea and vomiting. Chest pain and palpitations may also occur and patients frequently sweat a lot. MDMA is probably best known for its idiosyncratic effects of severe hyponatraemia leading to cerebral oedema, because a number of patients following the consumption of MDMA experience severe polydipsia.

Since there is no antidote treatment in MDMA overdose, the patients are managed with supportive measures. Hyperthermia should be treated with cooling packs and patients may require rapid cooling and administration of dantrolene. It is important to maintain good urine output in these patients with IV fluids as they are at risk of acute kidney injury. Metabolic acidosis is frequently present and can be managed with IV bicarbonate. Hypertension in these patients is best treated with calcium-channel blockers. If an arrhythmia develops, cardio-selective beta-blockers (e.g. metoprolol) can be given. Finally anxiety can be managed with benzodiazepines (e.g. diazepam).

4. What are the features of cocaine toxicity and how is it managed?
Cocaine can affect any system in the body but in overdose the systems more frequently affected are the cardiovascular and the central nervous systems. The cardiovascular effects result from increased adrenergic stimulation of the heart from reduced reuptake of catecholamines which can lead to various arrhythmias. Cocaine can also lead to an acute coronary syndrome as a result of coronary vasospasm as well as the rise in heart rate, blood pressure that leads to increased myocardial oxygen demand. In the central nervous system cocaine increases the risk of ischaemic and haemorrhagic stroke and can also induce seizures. Patients can also present with excited delirium, which puts them at an increased risk of sudden death. Finally cocaine can also lead to hyperthermia, rhabdomyolysis and acidosis.

Similarly to MDMA, there is no antidote to cocaine and cocaine toxicity should therefore be managed with supportive measures. Hypertension is best treated with dihydropyridine calcium channel blockers or nitrates. Beta blockers should be avoided as they may cause a paradoxical rise in blood pressure due to unopposed alpha stimulation. Arrhythmias can be managed with rate limiting calcium channel blockers (e.g. verapamil). Correction of acidosis with fluid resuscitation and IV HCO_3^- therapy may be useful in stabilising cardiomyocyte membranes and reducing the risk of arrhythmias. If an acute coronary syndrome is suspected the appropriate ACS protocol should be instigated.

Case 5 – **Carbon Monoxide and Cyanide Poisoning**

You are a Foundation Year 2 doctor working in the Emergency Department. A 35-year-old Livy Crossland was brought in by the ambulance crew, after firefighters found her collapsed in a house fire. She does not seem to have any evidence of burns or other injuries, however toxic fume inhalation is strongly suspected. She has been receiving high flow oxygen in the ambulance and has regained some consciousness although she still seems unwell. She has vomited twice in the ambulance.

Please conduct an A to E assessment of Ms Crossland and commence the initial management.

Latest observations:
HR: 130 BP: 80/40 RR: 25 SaO_2: 99 % (15 L of oxygen) Temp: 36.5 °C UO: unavailable

Danger

It is safe to approach the patient

Response

Patient responds to pain, it is appropriate to ask for help at this point

Airway

Look – no signs of burns or singes around the mouth or nostrils; there is no oedema in the airway; oxygen mask is fogging up as appropriate
Feel – trachea is central
Listen – normal breath sounds with no added upper airway sounds
Treat – patient is maintaining her own airway, monitor for signs of deterioration

Breathing

Look – does not appear cyanosed
Feel – chest expansion is symmetrical, resonant percussion
Listen – vesicular breath sounds are heard throughout
Measure – RR 25, SaO_2 on 15 L O_2 is 99 % via pulse oximetry
Treat – It is likely that the patient has carbon monoxide toxicity. High flow oxygen should therefore be continued via a tight fitting non-rebreathable mask with a reservoir bag
Reassess – regular ABGs should be taken to monitor SaO_2, % COHb and lactate

Further investigations:
- Perform an ABG - metabolic lactic acidosis
- Chest x-ray – normal
- % COHb is noted to be high at 15 %

Circulation

Look – patient looks pale, and peripherally shut down
Feel – patient feels cold to touch, pulse feels weak and thready
Listen – normal heart sounds
Measure – HR 130 BP 80/40, CRT = 4 s, temp 36.5 °C, UO: NA

Treat – the patient is profoundly hypotensive and tachycardic with end organ hypoperfusion and therefore requires aggressive fluid resuscitation (e.g. 500 ml of a crystalloid over 15 minutes). Up to 2000 ml of fluids can be given before escalation to inotropes. A urinary catheter should be inserted to monitor fluid balance.
Reassess – Blood pressure is not responsive to fluid therapy with features of fluid overload developing, features of end organ hypoperfusion persist.

Further investigations:
- ECG – demonstrates features in keeping with ischaemia with ST segment depression and T wave inversion across multiple leads
- Bloods (FBC, U&Es, LFT, clotting, troponin, pregnancy test)

As this patient is not responding to fluid therapy you should ask for senior help and consider starting inotropes such as norepinephrine, dobutamine, dopamine or isoprenaline depending on your hospital guidelines.

Disability

AVPU – patient is responsive to pain/GCS 8 (E2V3M3)
Capillary blood glucose - 7 mmol/L
Pupils – equal and reactive to light
Patient has increased tone in all 4 limbs with hyper-reflexia throughout and up going plantars bilaterally.

Patient exhibits features of multiple organ ischaemia as exhibited by CNS malfunction and cardiovascular instability. Because of the borderline GCS of 8, this patient may require intubation and ventilator support.

Exposure

- There is no evidence of any burns or trauma
- Abdomen is soft and non-tender, bowel sounds are present

Further investigations:
- Blood and urine toxicology screen
- Cyanide levels

Refer to Toxbase® for further information on various poisons and substances (https://www.toxbase.org). Your hospital should have the access details.

You should consider instigating empirical treatment for cyanide toxicity with hydroxycobalamin IV (vitamin B12).

Handover the patient to Dr Vishna (Critical care SpR)

Situation – This is Dr_____, the FY2 in A&E. I am calling regarding a 35-year-old female, Livy Crossland, who was brought in by ambulance after being found collapsed at a house fire. I suspect this patient has carbon monoxide and cyanide toxicity. However there is no evidence of burns.

Background – The patient was found collapsed by the firefighters at a house fire. She has received high flow oxygen whilst in the ambulance. She has slowly regained some consciousness since being extracted from the fire. No other past medical history is available at this point.

Assessment – She has not responded to a total of 2000 mL of fluid challenges with 0.9 % NaCl and her most recent observations are HR 130, BP 80/40, RR 25, SaO_2 98 % on 15 L O_2, temp 36.5 °C, urine output is low and she has a GCS of 8. The patient is peripherally shut down with evidence of end organ hypoperfusion and ischaemic ECG changes with ST depression and T wave inversion across multiple leads.

She has good air entry in both lungs but her blood gas shows a profound lactic acidosis, with a normal arterial alveolar gradient and SaO_2 85 %, COHb 15 %. Mobile chest X-ray showed no evidence of ARDS.

Her pupils are equal and reactive to light, but she has increased tone and brisk reflexes in all four limbs, as well as up-going plantars bilaterally. I have sent off bloods for cyanide levels and have continued treatment for carbon monoxide poisoning with high flow oxygen. I have also started empirical treatment for cyanide poisoning with IV hydroxycobalamin pending cyanide levels.

Recommendations – I would like you to come and urgently review this patient as I think she needs escalation of care. Is there anything else you would like me to do in the meantime?

Carbon monoxide and cyanide poisoning in brief

1. What is the pathophysiology of carbon monoxide and cyanide poisoning?
When dealing with toxic effects of smoke inhalation, one has to bear in mind that both carbon monoxide and cyanide are released from burning plastic. Both cause toxicity by depriving tissue of oxygen and impinging on aerobic metabolism. Carbon monoxide does this by reducing the oxygen carrying and dissociation ability of haemoglobin. Whilst cyanide prevents cells from utilising oxygen by blocking the mitochondrial electron transport chain. The effects of both are similar and predictable, with tissues that undergo high levels of aerobic metabolism being affected first.

These are namely the central nervous and cardiac tissues. Therefore poisoning with both substances will lead to confusion, drowsiness, seizures and coma, as well as cardiac ischaemia and cardiovascular instability.

2. What are the classical clinical features of carbon monoxide toxicity?
Carbon monoxide toxicity is more commonly seen due to faulty heaters and boilers, and as such, it mostly presents over the winter months. In mild toxicity the only symptoms maybe headaches, nausea, vomiting and fatigue. Several members of the household are usually affected and the symptoms disappear after leaving the premises. However, severe toxicity will lead to focal or generalised neurological deficits and cardiac ischaemia with arrhythmias leading to cardiovascular instability. Very severe toxicity may lead to skin blistering, pulmonary and cerebral oedema. However, the commonly mentioned 'cherry red complexion' is rarely seen in living patients.

3. What is the role of ABG sampling in carbon monoxide poisoning?
The arterial blood gas is the most crucial test in helping you diagnose carbon monoxide toxicity. Classically, it will show a lactic acidosis in the presence of normal oxygen tension and elevated % COHb. However bear in mind that in smokers the % COHb can be up to 10 %.

4. How do you manage carbon monoxide poisoning?
Carbon monoxide poisoning should be treated with high flow oxygen if the patient is able to maintain their airway and has a sufficient respiratory drive. If the airway or the respiratory drive are compromised, the patient should be intubated and ventilated with 100 % O_2. The use of hyperbaric O_2 treatment is controversial as the benefits are uncertain and it may not be readily available in all centres. It is important to perform a pregnancy test in all females of child bearing age as the foetus is much more vulnerable to the effects of carbon monoxide because of the higher affinity of foetal haemoglobin for carbon monoxide.

5. When should you suspect cyanide toxicity?
Cyanide toxicity occurs in house fires when plastic burns. It may also occur iatrogenically after a nitroprusside infusion. The clinical presentation is similar to carbon monoxide toxicity, although the history of exposure to toxic fumes is generally more obvious. On an arterial blood gas cyanide poisoning will cause a lactic acidosis with a normal oxygen tension and SaO_2, as it does not affect the oxygen-carrying ability of haemoglobin.

6. What are the key steps in the treatment of cyanide toxicity?
With regards to treatment, it is important to remove the source, whether it's contaminated clothing, ingested poisons or a nitroprusside infusion. Before any antidote is given, a blood sample must be sent for cyanide levels. There are several specific antidotes to cyanide, but the safest and most effective one following smoke inhalation is a hydroxycobalamin infusion. Other options include sodium nitrite or dicobalt edetate infusion. However, both have dangerous side effects and may worsen the patient's condition.

Orthopaedic Emergencies

Gerrard Gan

Septic Arthritis	252
Open Fracture	256
Acute Compartment Syndrome	262

Case 1 – **Septic Arthritis**

You are a Foundation Year 1 doctor working on the care of the elderly medicine ward. A nurse asks you to review an 85-year-old man with dementia, who is awaiting a nursing home placement. Since this morning he has developed fever with a painful left knee. He is a known diabetic, and has been ill with a respiratory tract infection over the past week. . The pain started today and has been getting progressively worse and has become intolerable despite painkillers. He is no longer able to bear weight on it. There is no history of injury.

Please conduct an A to E assessment of Mr Williams and commence the initial management.

Latest observations:

HR: 95 BP: 125/73 RR: 18 SaO_2: 98 % (room air) Temp: 38.3 °C UO: NA

Danger

It is safe to approach the patient.

Response

The patient is alert and responsive but in pain. Ensure analgesia is given.

Airway

The patient is talking. The airway is patent.

Breathing

Normal respiratory assessment

Circulation

Normal cardiovascular assessment, apart from a pyrexia of 38.3 °C

Disability

AVPU – Patient is alert and responsive/GCS 15
Check glucose – 11.2 mmol/L
Pupils – equal and reactive to light

Exposure

(Left Lower Limb - Knee)

It is noted that there is a wheelchair by the bedside and the patient is unable to ambulate due to pain.

Look – Knee is red and swollen. There is a pillow under the knee holding it in 20° flexion.
Feel – Warm. Notably tender. Large effusion.
Move – Restricted active and passive range of motion (10-30° of flexion) of the knee due to severe pain.
Tests – Unable to perform due to severe pain.

(Right Lower Limb - Knee)

Normal examination

On full exposure, there is no evidence of bleeding or rashes and the abdomen is soft and non-tender.

To finish off:
- Examine the joints above and below the affected joint
- Perform a brief neurovascular examination of the lower limbs

Further investigations:
- Bloods (FBC, CRP, urate, clotting, ESR)
- Blood cultures
- X-ray of the knee
- Joint aspirate for microscopy, culture, sensitivity and crystals

At this point you should suspect septic arthritis, with crystal arthropathies as a differential. Septic arthritis is an orthopaedic emergency, as the infection can destroy the joint within 24 hours. It requires urgent antibiotic treatment and an arthroscopic washout (see Box 1.)

Hand over the patient to Mr Shivani (Orthopaedics SpR)

Situation – This is Dr _____ the F1 in geriatrics. I have just seen Mr Williams, an 85-year-old gentleman, who I suspect has septic arthritis of his left knee.

Background – Mr Williams is an insulin dependent diabetic, who has been an inpatient for 1 week with a respiratory tract infection. He is currently awaiting a nursing home placement. Today he has developed a fever and a painful left knee, and the pain has been progressing despite painkillers.

Assessment – He has a pyrexia of 38.3. He is unable to weight-bear on his left leg. His left knee is red, hot and swollen. He has generalized tenderness and his range of motion is 10-30°. His right knee examination was normal. There is a large suprapatellar effusion. I have sent off bloods including FBC, CRP & cultures and ordered an X-ray.

Recommendation – I think this gentleman has septic arthritis of his left knee and I would like you to review him urgently to consider a joint aspiration and a washout, then to commence intravenous antibiotics. Is there anything you would like me to do in the meantime?

> **Box 1. Management of Septic Arthritis**
> 1) Nil by mouth & IV fluids
> 2) Adequate analgesia
> 3) Needle aspiration
> 4) Arthroscopic washout (sending cultures from washout)
> 5) Empirical antibiotics as per local guidelines (e.g. flucloxacillin or clindamycin)
> 6) Monitor with serial CRP measurements and clinical evaluation

Septic arthritis in brief:

1. What bacteria commonly cause septic arthritis?
- Staphylococcus aureus (commonest in adults)
- Streptococcus pneumonia, group B streptococci (S. pyogenes)
- Neisseria meningitidis and Neisseria gonorrhoeae (in young males with monoarthritis)
- Gram negative (e.g. Escherichia coli), more common in the elderly

2. What are the risk factors for septic arthritis?
- Pre-existing joint conditions (i.e. rheumatoid arthritis)
- Diabetes mellitus; immunosuppression; chronic kidney disease
- Recent joint surgery; prosthetic joints
- Intravenous drug use
- Age >80
- Joint steroid injections
- Concurrent systemic infection

3. What are the complications of septic arthritis?
- Rapid destruction of the joint with delayed treatment (>24 hrs)
- Osteomyelitis, skin and soft tissue infection
- Prosthesis failure
- Sepsis (which can be deadly)
- Degenerative joint disease and predisposition to osteoarthritis

4. What are the Kocher criteria for septic arthritis and when are they used?
In the paediatric population, Kocher criteria are useful to distinguish septic arthritis from transient synovitis of the hip.
1. Non weight-bearing
2. ESR > 40 mm/hr
3. WCC > 12
4. Pyrexia > 38.5°C

If positive: 1 criteria = 3% probability; 2 criteria = 40% probability; 3 criteria = 93% probability; 4 criteria = 99% probability of septic arthritis.

Case 2 – **Open Fracture**

You are a Foundation Year 2 doctor in emergency medicine. The triage nurse asked you to review an 82-year-old lady, Mrs Roberts, who presented to A&E with an open right tibial fracture following a fall at home. She had missed a step and fell down 2 steps. She denies any other injuries.

Please conduct an A to E assessment of Mrs Roberts and commence the initial management.

Latest observations:
HR: 105 BP: 100/73 RR: 16 SaO$_2$: 98 % (RA) Temp: 36.9 °C UO: NA

Danger

There is blood-soaked bandage on her right leg and a velcro splint. Wear an apron and gloves.

Response

The patient is alert and responsive but in pain. Administer strong analgesia.

Airway

The patient is talking. There is no suspicion of head or neck injury.

Breathing

Normal respiratory assessment

Circulation

Look – pale, dry mucous membranes
Feel – cool and clammy, rapid pulse with reduced volume, reduced skin turgor
Listen – normal heart sounds
Measure – HR: 105 BP: 100/73 CRT 4 s UO: NA
Treat – obtain IV access and commence intravenous fluid resuscitation
Reassess – HR: 85 BP: 115/78 CRT 2 secs

Disability

AVPU – Patient is alert and responsive/GCS 15 (E4, V5, M6)
Check glucose – 4.7 mmol/L
Pupils – equal and reactive to light

Exposure

(Right Lower Limb)

The leg is in a padded splint with velcro straps across the front. There is a blood-soaked bandage at mid tibial level. Continue the assessment with gloves and apron.

Look – after ensuring adequate analgesia, the velcro is opened at the front, leaving the splint in situ (dressing removed). There is an obvious varus deformity along the tibia. There is a bleeding 2cm wound with a bony protrusion on the medial aspect of the right leg.

Feel – the lower leg is very tender. The foot is cold to touch and the pulses are impalpable. Sensation is intact and the compartments are soft.
Move – Active and passive range of motion of the right leg are not performed due to pain and deformity.

No neurological deficit distal to the injury.

(Left Lower Limb)

Normal

On full exposure, there is no evidence of rashes and the abdomen is soft and non-tender.

To finish off:
- Keep the patient nil by mouth
- Prescribe analgesia

Further investigations:
- Bloods (FBC, U&E, clotting screen)
- Group & Save
- Radiography of the injured limb
- Broad spectrum antibiotics as per British Orthopaedic Association Guidelines (within 3 hours). Co-amoxiclav or Cefuroxime, and continue until wound debridement (Clindamycin if penicillin allergic).
- Repeat neurovascular examinations regularly.
- Medical photography of the wound.
- Cover in saline soaked gauze and impermeable film to prevent desiccation.

This patient has an open fracture. Open fractures are orthopaedic emergencies, as there is a high risk of infection. Furthermore, this patient has compromised blood supply to her right lower limb. It requires urgent vascular repair, debridement and fixation of the fracture as well as antibiotics and tetanus prophylaxis.

Hand over the patient to Mr Shivani (Orthopaedics SpR)

Situation – This is Dr _____ the F2 in A&E. I have just seen Mrs Roberts, an 82-year-old lady, who has on open fracture of her right tibia with compromised distal blood supply.

Background – Mrs Roberts fell at home from a height of 2 steps.

Assessment – On initial assessment she was alert with a GCS of 15, with no head or neck injuries. She was clinically hypovolaemic. She is wearing a Velcro splint applied by the paramedics. However on gently removing this, she has an obvious varus deformity, and a 2 cm wound on the medial side. Her dorsalis pedis and posterior tibial pulses were impalpable and the foot was cold to touch. Distal neurological function was intact. Her left leg examination was normal.

Recommendation – This lady has an open fracture of her right tibia with compromised distal blood supply and I would like you to review her urgently. She is nil by mouth. I have ordered X-ray and bloods. I have irrigated the wound and covered it with saline-soaked gauze and an impermeable dressing. I have given her a dose of co-amoxiclav. Is there anything else you would like me to do?

> If the tetanus immunisation history is unknown or incomplete the patient, depending on the levels of contamination, should receive prophylaxis (vaccine or vaccine with an immunoglobulin). If the vaccination course has been completed but the last dose was more than 5 years ago, the patient should still receive a tetanus vaccine.

Open fractures in brief:

1. What is the management of open fractures?
- Nil by mouth and fluid resuscitation if large volume of blood loss
- Adequate analgesia (e.g. IV morphine) with an anti-emetic
- IV Antibiotics (as per local guidelines)
- Cover the wound with sterile saline soaked gauze
- Immobilise the fractured limb
- Immediate surgical intervention to restore the blood flow
- Debride the wound, reduce and stabilise the fracture
- Tetanus prophylaxis

2. What are the complications of open fractures?
- Bleeding
- Neurovascular injury
- Compartment syndrome
- Bone and soft tissue infection (including tetanus)
- Non-union/malunion
- Amputation

Case 3 – **Acute Compartment Syndrome**

You are a Foundation Year 1 doctor working in Trauma & Orthopaedics. The ward nurse asks you to review a 32-year-old gentleman, Mr Jones, who had a tibial nailing operation 2 days ago for a closed tibial fracture. He is complaining of severe and worsening pain despite analgesia.

Please conduct an A to E assessment of Mr Jones and commence the initial management.

Latest observations:
HR: 105 BP: 125/80 RR: 16 SaO$_2$: 99 % (RA) Temp: 36.7 °C UO: NA

Danger
It is safe to approach the patient.

Response
The patient is alert and responsive.

Airway
The patient is talking.

Breathing
Normal respiratory assessment

Circulation
Tachycardia (HR 105), otherwise unremarkable

Disability
AVPU – Patient is alert and responsive/GCS 15
Check glucose – 4.8 mmol/L
Pupils – equal and reactive to light

Exposure
(Left Lower Limb – Leg)

Following a brief discussion with your seniors the backslab on his left leg should be completely removed.

Look – the leg is swollen below the knee. The knee is held flexed at 20° and the ankle is plantar flexed.
Feel – cool and exceptionally tender throughout. Distal pulses are weakly palpable. CRT 5 sec . Calf is tense.
Move – Any passive extension of the knee or dorsiflexion of the ankle causes severe pain.
Tests – Passive stretch test positive (increase in pain levels on stretching of the ischaemic compartment)

(Right Lower Limb – Leg)
Normal

On full exposure, there is no evidence of bleeding or rashes and the abdomen is soft and non-tender.

Further investigations:
- Bloods (FBC, U&E, clotting screen, d-dimer, creatinine kinase)
- Consider intra-compartmental pressure study if unsure of the diagnosis

> At this point you should suspect a compartment syndrome, with deep vein thrombosis as a differential. Compartment syndrome is an orthopaedic emergency, as the hypoxic tissue can undergo irreversible damage within 6 – 8 hours. It requires the removal of the cast, bandages and dressings, before considering an emergent fasciotomy (see Box 1).

Hand over the patient to Mr Shivani (Orthopaedics SpR)

Situation – This is Dr _____ the F1 in Trauma & Orthopaedics. I have just seen Mr Jones, a 32-year-old gentleman, who I suspect has compartment syndrome of his left lower leg.

Background – Mr Jones was admitted with a left tibial fracture 3 days ago. He underwent tibial nailing 2 days ago. Mr Jones has been managing well until this morning, when he developed worsening pain in his left leg despite his painkillers.

Assessment – On initial assessment he appeared clinically well but was complaining of severe pain in his left lower leg. Removing his plaster cast completely, his left leg appeared pale and swollen below the knee. His calf was tense. His distal pulses were weakly palpable, and his CRT was 5 sec. His range of motion was severely restricted due to pain, and the passive stretch test was positive (dorsiflexing his toes and ankle causes severe pain). His right leg examination was normal.

Recommendation – I think this gentleman has a compartment syndrome of his left leg and I would like you to review him urgently to consider compartment pressure testing or a fasciotomy. Is there anything you would like me to do in the meantime?

> **Box 1. Management of compartment syndrome**
> - Nil by mouth and intravenous fluids
> - Adequate analgesia (e.g. IV morphine)
> - Removal of casts, bandages and dressing from limb (split to skin)
> - Elevate the limb
> - Consider intra-compartmental pressure study
> - Consider fasciotomy

Compartment syndrome in brief:

1. What is the pathogenesis of compartment syndrome?
- Insult/Injury
- Bleeding and soft tissue swelling occurs in a compartment bounded by fascia
- Intra-compartmental pressure increases
- Decrease of venous and lymphatic return
- Intra-compartmental pressure exceeds diastolic blood pressure
- Blood circulation is cut off
- Oxygen sensitive tissues (ie. muscle and nerves) undergo ischaemia changes
- Tissue necrosis ensues
- Triggers an inflammatory response, causing further swelling in the compartment

2. What are the features of compartment syndrome?

EARLY (3 PS)	LATE (3 PS)
Pain (out of proportion to injury)	Perishingly cold
Pallor	Pulselessness
Paraesthesiae	Paralysis

3. How is a compartment syndrome diagnosed?
Compartment syndrome is a clinical diagnosis. Investigations such as intra-compartmental pressure studies will help confirm the diagnosis and guide management. If the absolute pressure is >30 mmHg or within 30mm of diastolic blood pressure, the study is positive and is an indication for an urgent fasciotomy.

4. What are the complications of a compartment syndrome?
- Rhabdomyolysis
- Renal failure
- Volkmann's ischaemic contractures
- Limb amputation

Obstetric and Gynaecological Emergencies

Ruoxing Du

Adnexal Torsion	268
Ectopic Pregnancy	272
Antepartum Haemorrhage	276
Pre-Eclampsia	280
Postpartum Haemorrhage	284

Case 1 – **Adnexal Torsion**

You are a Foundation Year 2 doctor working in Emergency Medicine. You have been asked to see Miss Wallis, a 23-year-old lady. The triage nurse tells you that she presents with severe lower abdominal pain, which started whilst playing a rugby match. She has also been feeling very nauseous and has been vomiting. The patient is not sexually active and has a past medical history of polycystic ovary syndrome, for which she takes the oral contraceptive pill.

Please conduct an A to E assessment of Miss Wallis and commence the initial management.

Latest observations
HR: 109 BP: 100/70 RR: 20 SaO_2: 98 % (RA) Temp: 37.1 °C UO: NA

Danger
It is safe to approach the patient.

Response
Patient is responsive, but moans in pain.

Airway
The patient is talking in full sentences, and the airway is patent.

Breathing
Look – equal chest wall expansion, no use of accessory muscles
Feel – trachea is central, symmetrical chest movement, resonant to percussion
Listen – vesicular breath sounds
Measure – RR 20; SaO_2 98 % on room air
Treat – continuously monitor oxygen saturation using pulse oximetry. Aim for target oxygen saturations of 94 – 98 %

Circulation
Look – pale, peripheral cyanosis, JVP not visible, no oedema
Feel – warm peripheries, regular rapid pulse with normal volume
Listen – normal heart sounds
Measure – HR 109, BP 100/70, CRT 1 second, temp 37.1 °C, UO: NA
Treat – obtain IV access, commence fluids, give paracetamol and cyclizine for pain and nausea (consider stronger analgesia e.g. morphine)
Reassess – HR 98, BP 110/80, patient is now feeling more comfortable

Disability
AVPU – alert/GCS15
Blood glucose – 4.7 mmols
Pupils – equal and reactive to light

Exposure

Abdominal examination reveals rebound tenderness and guarding localized in the left iliac fossa.

Ensure the patient is nil by mouth for now.

Further investigations:
- Urine beta-HCG should be tested on all females with abdominal pain of a child-bearing age. This is negative in her case.
- Bloods (FBC, U&E, LFT, clotting studies, amylase, group and save)
- Venous blood gas to quickly assess pH, Hb and lactate levels
- Urine dipstick to look for signs of infection, blood or glucose. This is normal in her case
- Transvaginal or abdominal ultrasound if available to look for the cause of pain

Hand over the patient to Mr Seah (Gynaecology SpR)

Situation – Dr Seah, I am _____ the FY2 doctor working in A&E. I want to refer a 23-year-old lady, Alice Wallis, who presented with sudden onset abdominal pain 2 hours ago. I am concerned that she may have adnexal torsion.

Background – She is currently not sexually active, and has a past medical history of PCOS, controlled by the oral contraceptive pill. This pain started two hours ago, with associated nausea and vomiting, whilst playing sports..

Assessment – On examination, she is very tender over the left iliac fossa. She is currently haemodynamically stable and afebrile. Her urinary pregnancy test and dipstick are negative. She now has IV access, and I have taken bloods and given her fluids.

Recommendation – My impression is that she has adnexal torsion. Would you be able to review her as soon as possible? I will keep her nil by mouth until then. Please let me know if there is anything else you want me to do for her in the mean time.

Adnexal torsion in brief

1. What are some of the other differential diagnoses to consider in this patient?
Gynaecological causes:
- Ovarian cyst accident including torsion, haemorrhage, cyst rupture
- PID/tubo-ovarian abscess
- Ectopic pregnancy

Surgical causes:
- Renal colic
- Appendicitis

2. What is ovarian torsion?
Ovarian torsion is the twisting of the ovary, and sometimes the fallopian tube, around their vascular pedicle, otherwise known as adnexal torsion. The twisting first obstructs venous outflow, leading to oedema and engorgement. This swelling eventually causes the arterial blood flow to become compromised, leading to ischaemia and infarction of the ovaries. It is more common during reproductive years, especially in patients with known ovarian cysts, polycystic ovarian syndrome, ovarian hyper-stimulation or long ovarian ligaments.

3. How do you diagnose ovarian torsion?
It is mostly a diagnosis based on clinical findings. Pelvic ultrasound may show unilateral enlargement of the ovary, where the ovarian stroma appears oedamatous and the follicles are peripherally placed, often with free fluid in the pelvis. Occasionally, there may be a co-existing adnexal mass. Colour or power Doppler is rarely useful but may demonstrate reduced blood flow. A CT scan is generally not useful in the assessment of pelvic pathology but may help to assess for other abnormalities e.g. appendicitis or nephrocalcinosis.

The definitive diagnosis can only be made during a laporoscopy/ laparotomy. Therefore early referral to a gynaecologist is important.

4. What are the treatment options for an ovarian torsion?
Early laparoscopic management is crucial. This involves surgical de-torsion and leaving the ovary in place following the detorsion, even if it appears dusky blue or black. It has been shown that in most cases, ovarian function is preserved.

Follow up may be required to assess ovarian function post-operatively.

If an ovarian cyst is identified, it may require surgery at a later date. Post-menopausal women with torsion should be managed with bilateral oophorectomy.

Case 2 – **Ectopic Pregnancy**

You are a Foundation Year 2 doctor working in the Emergency Department. You have been asked to see Miss Whittle, a 24-year-old lady, who has been suffering from worsening abdominal pain for the last few hours. Her last period was 8 weeks ago.

Please conduct an A to E assessment of Miss Whittle and commence the initial management.

Latest observations

HR: 120 BP: 86/63 RR: 20 SaO_2: 98 % (RA) Temp: 37.1 °C UO: NA

Danger
It is safe to approach the patient.

Response
Patient is responsive, but moans in pain.

Airway
Airway is clear (patient is talking in full sentences).

Breathing
Look – equal chest expansion, no use of accessory muscles
Feel – trachea is central, symmetrical chest movement, resonant percussion
Listen – vesicular breath sounds
Measure – RR 20; SaO_2 98 % on room air.
Treat – monitor oxygen saturations. Aim for oxygen saturations of 94 – 98 %.

Circulation
Look – pale, peripheral cyanosis, JVP not visible, no oedema
Feel – cool peripheries, regular rapid pulse with reduced volume
Listen – normal heart sounds
Measure – HR 120, BP 86/63, capillary refill 4 seconds, UO: NA, temp 37.1 °C
Treat – obtain IV access and give a fluid challenge of 500 mL 0.9 % sodium chloride. Aim to maintain the patient's blood pressure to >100/80 mmHg.
Reassess – patient's blood pressure is now 110/80 mmHg

Disability
AVPU – responsive to voice/GCS13 (E4V4M5)
Blood glucose – 4.5 mmols
Pupils – equal and reactive to light

Exposure
Abdominal examination reveals a tender abdomen with guarding, particularly in the left iliac fossa

Further investigations:
- Urine pregnancy test (positive in her case)
- Blood tests: FBC, U&E, LFT, clotting screen, beta-HCG and cross match

Hand over the patient to Dr Smith (Gynaecology SpR)

Situation – Good afternoon Dr Smith, I am_____ the FY2 doctor working in A&E. I have a 24 year old Miss Whittle, who I suspect has an ectopic pregnancy.

Background – Her last menstrual period was 8 weeks ago and she is currently sexually active.

Assessment – She is haemodynamically unstable, with a blood pressure of 86/63mmHg, heart rate of 120. She is apyrexial and maintaining normal oxygen saturation. Her urine pregnancy test is positive. On examination, there is abdominal guarding, and the abdomen is particularly tender over the left iliac fossa.

Recommendation – There is a high suspicion of an ectopic pregnancy, and given that she is haemodynamically unstable, please can you come and review her urgently. I have taken bloods and started IV fluid resuscitation. I will keep her nil by mouth until you assess her. Is there anything else you want me to do for her in the meantime?

Box 1. Management of ectopic pregnancy
1. Resuscitation - ensure patient is haemodynamically stable. If she isn't then urgent fluid resuscitation with crystalloid fluid should be commenced and an urgent request for cross match of 4 units of red blood cells should be sent.
2. Urgent gynaecology specialist assessment and triage.
3. If the patient is haemodynamically stable, it is reasonable to carry out further investigations, including serum beta-hCG and transvaginal ultrasound to determine the location of the pregnancy.

Ectopic pregnancy in brief:

1. What is an ectopic pregnancy?
Ectopic pregnancy occurs when a fertilised ovum implants outside of the uterus. The most common site is in the fallopian tubes (93-95%). The other locations include:
- Cervix
- Interstitial
- Cornual
- Ovary
- Abdomen
- Caesarean scar

Patients typically present at less than 6 weeks gestation. The common presentation will be a woman with abdominal pain +/- light vaginal bleeding with a history of missed menstrual period.

The danger with ectopic pregnancy is the risk of rupture as the foetus grows in size, leading to haemorrhage within the abdomen. Thus early detection and management is vital.

2. What are the risk factors that make ectopic pregnancy more likely?
- Previous sexually transmitted infections (chlamydia, gonorrhoea)
- Intrauterine contraceptive devices
- Damaged fallopian tubes, from salpingitis, previous surgery
- Endometriosis
- Previous ectopic pregnancy
- Pregnancy after tubal ligation

It is important to remember that most women with ectopic pregnancy don't have any risk factors. Thus it is vital for all women of child bearing age presenting with abdominal pain to have an urinary pregnancy test.

Case 3 – **Antepartum Haemorrhage**

You are a Foundation Year 2 doctor working in the maternity triage unit. You have been asked to attend to a patient, Mrs. Johnson. She is a 30 year old lady who is currently 34 weeks pregnant. She tells you that her pregnancy so far has been uneventful. Today, she presents with mild vaginal bleeding, which started 5 hours ago and she is now feeling very faint and worried.

Please conduct an A to E assessment of Mrs Johnson and commence the initial management.

Latest observations
HR: 120 BP: 86/53 RR: 26 SaO_2: 96 % (RA) Temp: 36.9 °C UO: NA

Danger

Safe to approach the patient, but wear apron and gloves.

Response

Patient is responsive. Perform left lateral tilt with the use of a wedge, bed or clothing, before further assessment. This ensures uterine displacement to ensure better cardiac return via the inferior vena cava.

You may want to call for additional help whilst you proceed with a quick ABCDE assessment.

Airway

Airway is clear (patient is talking in full sentences).

Breathing

Look – patient is breathing rapidly. There is equal chest wall expansion, no use of accessory muscles. No peripheral or central cyanosis.
Feel – trachea is central, symmetrical chest movement, resonant to percussion
Listen – vesicular breath sounds
Measure – RR 26; SaO$_2$ 96 % (RA)
Treat – move on

Circulation

Look – pale
Feel – cool peripheries, regular rapid pulse with reduced volume
Listen – normal heart sounds
Measure – HR 120 bpm, BP 86/53 mmHg, CRT 3 seconds, Temp: 36.9°C UO: NA
Treat – insert 2 large-bore cannulae (16G), initiate fluid resuscitation (e.g. up to 2L fluid challenge in 500mL boluses).
Reassess – HR 100 bpm, BP rises to 100/70

Disability

AVPU – alert/GCS 15
Blood glucose – 4.5 mmols
Pupils – equal and reactive to light

Exposure

Abdominal examination reveals a tender and tense uterus. There is a soaked pad on observation. Do not perform vaginal examination if you suspect placenta previa.

During antenatal haemorrhage CTG should be used to monitor foetal wellbeing. The labour ward and the anaesthetists should be notified immediately for the possible emergency delivery of the baby. The patient's rhesus status should be checked and if she is rhesus-negative, she will need to be given prophylactic anti-D immunoglobulin.

Recognition of major obstetric haemorrhage
It is vital to identify that this is a major obstetric haemorrhage (MOH) and requires an urgent MOH call via 2222.

Further investigations:
- Blood (FBC, U&E, LFT, clotting studies, group and save)
- VBG might be beneficial as you can obtain vital information including Hb level
- CTG if available
- Contact blood bank for urgent cross match and urgent transfusion

As this is a major obstetric emergency, keep the handover brief to the obstetrician.

Hand over the patient to Dr Newton (Obstetrics SpR)

Situation – This is a 30 year old lady, 34 weeks pregnant, who has a major antepartum haemorrhage.

Background – The vaginal bleeding has been on going for the last 5 hours.

Assessment – She is very haemodynamically unstable, with a tender abdomen and tense uterus.

Recommendation – I have started intravenous fluids and have requested an urgent 4 units cross match of red blood cells. We have transferred her to the labour ward. She is NBM and we have commenced continuous electronic foetal monitoring (CTG). Please could you kindly review her urgently. Is there anything else you would like me to do in the meantime?

Antepartum haemorrhage in brief

1. What are the differentials for antepartum haemorrhage?
- Placental abruption
- Placenta praevia
- Uterine rupture
- Vasa praevia

2. What is placental abruption?
Placental abruption is the premature separation of the placenta from the uterus. Care is needed in managing these patients, because despite minimal visible blood loss there may be a large internal haemorrhage. There is an increased risk of recurrence in future pregnancies.

3. What are the consequences of placental abruption?
There is increased morbidity and mortality to both the foetus and the mother. The foetus may develop brain anoxia from placental insufficiency, which can quickly lead to brain damage and death. The mother can go on to develop hypovolaemic shock from severe blood loss with all its related complications. These patients are also at risk of severe postpartum haemorrhage.

4. How to distinguish placental abruption from placenta praevia?
In placenta praevia the placenta lies in the lower segment of the uterus, which may or may not be covering the cervical os. It generally tends to be more dangerous for the mother than the foetus. It is also important to note that women with placenta praevia are also at risk of placental abruption.

The table below describes the main differences in presentation between placental abruption and placenta praevia.

PLACENTAL ABRUPTION	PLACENTA PRAEVIA
• shock may be out of proportion to visible blood loss • constant pain • tender and tense uterus • normal lie and presentation • foetal heart rate: absent/distressed • co-existing coagulopathy is common	• shock is in proportion to visible blood loss • painless bleeding • non-tender uterus • lie and presentation may be abnormal • foetal heart rate usually normal • co-existing coagulopathy is rare

Case 4 – **Pre-eclampsia**

You are a Foundation Year 2 doctor working with the Obstetrics & Gynaecology on-call team. You have been called to attend to a patient, Mrs Simmons, a 38 year old lady at maternity triage. She is 36 weeks pregnant, and is complaining of a severe headache and visual disturbances.

Please conduct an A to E assessment of Mrs Simmons and commence the initial management.

Latest observations

HR: 90 BP: 170/113 RR: 16 SaO$_2$: 99 % (RA) Temp: 36.9 °C UO: NA

Danger

Safe to approach the patient

Response

Patient is responsive but is confused.

Airway

Airway is clear (patient is talking in full sentences)

Breathing

Look – equal chest expansion, no use of accessory muscles
Feel – trachea is central, symmetrical chest movement, resonant percussion
Listen – vesicular breath sounds
Measure – RR 16; SaO$_2$ 99 % on room air
Treat – continuously monitor oxygen saturation using pulse oximetry. Aim for oxygen saturations of 94 – 98 %

Circulation

Look – pale, no cyanosis, JVP not visible, no oedema
Feel – warm peripheries, regular pulse with normal volume and character
Listen – normal heart sounds
Measure – HR 90, BP 170/113, CRT 1 seconds, UO: NA
Treat – ensure patient is in left lateral tilt, obtain IV access. Start oral labetalol immediately to manage blood pressure and continue monitoring.

Disability

AVPU – alert/GCS14 (E4V4M6)
Blood glucose – 6.5 mmols
Pupils – equal and reactive to light

Exposure

Abdominal examination reveals a tender RUQ. The foetal head is engaged. She has bilateral oedematous leg and ankles.

Further investigations:
- Blood (FBC, U&E, LFT, clotting, blood glucose, urate)
- Urine dipstick to look for proteinuria (3+++ in her case)
- Catheterise to measure urine output and collect 24 hour urine to measure protein levels
- CTG monitoring to monitor foetal wellbeing

Hand over the patient to Dr Woodman (Obstetrics SpR)

Situation – Hello, I am _____ , the FY2 doctor working in maternity triage. I would like to refer a 36 week pregnant lady, who has severe pre-eclampsia.

Background - She is complaining of a severe headache and visual disturbances.

Assessment – Her current observations are: HR: 90 BP: 170/113 RR: 16 and SaO2: 99 % on room air. Her blood glucose was 6.5. Her urine dip revealed 3+ protein. On examination, she has a tender right upper quadrant, bilateral pitting oedema. We have sent off blood tests, and are awaiting results.

Recommendation - I think this lady has severe pre-eclampsia. I have given her labetolol stat and have started her on regular oral labetolol. She will need a repeat BP check to see if she responds. I have transferred her to the labour ward for further monitoring and assessment and have made her NBM. Please let me know what else you would like me to do in the meantime.

Pre-eclampsia and eclampsia in brief

1. What is pre-eclampsia?
Pre-eclampsia is new hypertension presenting after 20 weeks gestation with significant proteinuria.
It is diagnosed based on the following factors:
- New hypertension found after 20 weeks gestation (BP>140/90mmHg)
- Significant proteinuria (use either 24 hour urine protein (> 300mg) or urinary protein:creatinine ratio > 30mg/mmol)

2. How is pre-eclampsia managed?
Pre-eclampsia is managed by:
- Managing hypertension with oral anti-hypertensives
- Close monitoring of maternal blood tests including full blood count, renal function, liver function and clotting to check for complications of pre-eclampsia.
- Monitoring of foetal well being with CTG and regular ultrasound scans for foetal growth as there may be a co-existing foetal growth restriction.
- Aim for delivery at 37 weeks gestation. Women with pre-eclampsia have a higher risk of needing pre-term delivery as a result of their condition, in which case a course of antenatal corticosteroids may be required to aid foetal lung maturation.

3. What are the complications of pre-eclampsia?
- Eclampsia
- HELLP syndrome
- Renal failure
- Pulmonary oedema
- VTE (PE/DVT)

Eclampsia is a convulsive condition associated with pre-eclampsia. This is a life-threatening condition that requires urgent management. Be aware that women can still develop eclampsia within 48 hours post delivery.

HELLP syndrome is haemolysis, elevated liver enzymes and low platelet count.

	MEANING	CLINICAL FINDINGS
H	Haemolysis	Dark urine, raised LDH, anaemia
EL	Elevated liver enzymes	Epigastric pain, abnormal clotting, liver failure
LP	low platelets	Normally self-limiting

Case 5 – **Post-partum Haemorrhage**

You are a Foundation Year 2 doctor working on the labour ward. A midwife just shouted at you to come and assess Mrs Kumar, a 31 year old lady. She is having heavy vaginal bleeding 30 minutes after a delivery of a 4.3kg baby boy via forceps delivery.

Please conduct an A to E assessment of Mrs Kumar and commence the initial management.

Latest observations

HR: 120 BP: 87/54 RR: 23 SaO$_2$: 98 % (RA) temp: 36.9 °C UO: NA

Danger

Safe to approach the patient but it is important to wear gloves and an apron.

Response

The patient is responsive but appears drowsy.

> The patient has just delivered and is bleeding significantly. This is a post-partum haemorrhage (PPH). The immediate thing to do is to call the buzzer to alert the team and ask for help:
> MOA(N)S
> - Midwife
> - Obstetrican (senior)
> - Anaesthetist
> - Scribe
>
> (N = neonatologist, who you don't need in this case)
>
> You can proceed to ABCDE assessment once you have called for help.

Airway

Airway is clear

Breathing

Look – equal chest wall expansion, no use of accessory muscles
Feel – trachea is central, symmetrical chest movement, resonant percussion
Listen – vesicular breath sounds
Measure – RR 23; SaO_2 98 % on room air
Treat – continuously monitor oxygen saturation using pulse oximetry. Aim for target oxygen saturations of 94 – 98 %.

Circulation

Look – pale, peripheral cyanosis, JVP not visible, no oedema
Feel – cool peripheries, regular rapid pulse with reduced volume
Listen – normal heart sounds
Measure – HR 120, BP 87/54 mmHg, CRT 3 seconds, UO: NA
Treat – lie patient flat, catheterize her and ask for your midwife to help you ensure IV access, start fluid resuscitation and contact blood bank for an urgent cross match. Insert a urinary catheter to monitor fluid balance.
Reassess - maintain the patient's blood pressure to above 100/70 mmHg

Disability

AVPU – alert/ GCS 15
Blood glucose – 4.5 mmols
Pupils – equal and reactive to light

Exposure

Vaginal examination reveals estimated blood loss of 1200mL. There are some blood clots around the cervical os. You cannot see any evidence of perineal trauma.

> Vaginal examination is vital here, which looks for:
> - Uterine inversion
> - Removal of clots from the cervix and uterus that may have collected, which will improve uterine tone.
> - Identify any local trauma to the perineum causing the bleed.
> - If you suspect uterine atony as the main cause, then you should start bimanual uterine compression.

Consider administering uterotonics e.g. syntocinon infusion, ergometrine or misoprostol.

If bleeding exceeds 1500mls and is on-going, then a Major Obstetric Haemorrhage call needs to be put out.

Hand over to Dr Newton (Obstetrics SpR)

Situation –This is Mrs Kumar, who is having a postpartum haemorrhage.

Background – She delivered a 4.3kg boy 30 minutes ago with complete delivery of the placenta .

Assessment – Her BP is 87/54 and HR is 120. The estimated blood loss is 1200mL. She is catheterized and the midwife has started uterine massage.

Recommendation - I suspect uterine atony. Please let me know how I can help you.

> Box 1. Estimated blood loss- up to 1000ml can be managed with basic measures:
> - Close monitoring
> - IV access
> - Bloods (FBC and Group and Save)
>
> Identify possible causes of PPH (listed below). Most cases of PPH have NO identifiable risk factors.
>
> Management of moderate/severe PPH
> 1. Call for help
> 2. Empty bladder (catheterise), uterine massage, IV fluids and controlled cord traction if the placenta has not yet been delivered
> 3. Uterotonic drugs
> - 1st line drugs: Oxytocin or Ergometrine or combined Syntometrine
> - 2nd line drugs: repeat bolus of above, Misoprostol, Oxytocin infusion or Carboprost IM
> 4. If the above fails, then consider examination under anaesthesia (EUA)
> - If suspected uterine atony, consider uterine balloon tamponade
> - If patient remains unstable, consider uterine artery embolisation, laparotomy followed by either B Lynch suture, internal artery ligation or hysterectomy.

Post-partum haemorrhage in brief:

1. What is the definition of primary post-partum haemorrhage (PPH)?
Primary PPH occurs within 24 hours of delivery. It is defined as a loss of more than 500mls of blood during vaginal delivery and more than 1000mls within the first 24 hours of delivery.

2. What are some of the causes of primary PPH?
　　Remember it as the 4Ts
　　• Tone - atony. This accounts for 80 % of cases. More common with prolonged labour, grand multiparity, over-distension of the uterus (polyhydramnios and multiple pregnancies) and fibroids.
　　• Trauma - uterine rupture, cervical tear, high vaginal tear, perineal trauma.
　　• Tissue - retained placenta or part of the placenta.
　　• Thrombin (coagulopathy - rare): congenital disorders, anticoagulant therapy or disseminated intravascular coagulopathy (DIC).

Paediatric Emergencies

Samuel Quek and Sana Owais Subhan

Anaphylaxis	290
Testicular Torsion	294
Acute Appendicitis	298
Non-Accidental Injury	302
Exacerbation of Asthma in a Child	306
Paediatric Basic Life Support	312
Upper Airway Obstruction	316

Case 1 – **Anaphylaxis**

You are the on call Foundation Year 1 doctor working in paediatrics. You have been asked by one of the nurses to urgently review James Bennett, a five-year-old boy. He was just started on co-amoxiclav for a suspected chest infection and has suddenly developed difficulty breathing, an erythematous rash, and swelling of his tongue and mouth.

Please conduct an A to E assessment of James Bennett and commence the initial management.

Latest observations:
HR: 130 BP: 90/60, RR: 32, SaO_2 90 % (RA), Temp 36.7 °C UO: NA

Danger
It is safe to approach the patient

Response
Patient is crying

Airway
Immediately stop any potential causes of anaphylaxis (in this case IV antibiotics)
Look – swollen lips and tongue, rash around the mouth and cheeks
Listen – raspy breaths, stridor
Treat – call for senior help immediately and ask for intramuscular adrenaline
Reassess – move on

Breathing
Look – use of accessory muscles, intercostal recession
Feel – central trachea, uniformly reduced chest expansion and percussion
Listen – noisy breathing, stridor but equal and good air entry
Measure – RR 32, Sats 90 % (on room air).
Treat – high flow oxygen (15 L of 100 %) via a non-rebreathe mask. Continuously monitor SaO_2 for deterioration. Consider bronchodilator therapy if there is respiratory deterioration.
Reassess – RR 29, SaO_2 99 % (15L O_2)

Circulation
Look – pale, sweaty, flushed
Feel – warm to touch
Listen – normal heart sounds
Measure – HR 130, BP 90/60, CRT <2 seconds, Temp 36.7 °C, UO: not available
Treat – Obtain IV access. Administer intramuscular adrenaline, and chlorphenamine and hydrocortisone intravenously.
Reassess – HR 110, BP 108/70, RR 25, Temp 36.7 °C

Disability

AVPU – Alert/GCS 15
Blood glucose – 5.3 mmol/L
Pupils – equal and reactive to light

Exposure

There is an erythematous rash on the chest and arms. The abdomen is soft and non-tender.

Hand over patient to Dr Brown (Paediatrics SpR)

Situation – Hello Dr Brown, this is _____ , the FY1 in paediatrics. I am calling you regarding James Bennett, a five year old boy, who has just had an anaphylactic reaction.

Background – He was started on co-amoxiclav for a suspected chest infection and has developed signs of an anaphylactic reaction.

Assessment – On assessment, he was tearful, pale and sweaty. He had visible swelling of his lips and tongue as well as a rash around his mouth, chest and on his arms. He was tachypnoeic with a RR of 32 and saturations of 90% on room air. I treated him with high flow oxygen via a non-rebreathe mask and IM adrenaline, chlorphenamine and hydrocortisone. He has significantly improved following the administration of adrenaline and the swelling has subsided.

Recommendation – I would appreciate it if you could come and review James. In the meantime, is there anything else you would like me to do?

Anaphylaxis in brief

1. What is anaphylaxis?
Anaphylaxis is a life-threatening reaction to an agent, such as food, medication or insect stings. It occurs in people previously exposed to a particular antigen to which they have developed IgE antibodies. When a repeat exposure occurs, the preformed IgE antibodies bind to mast cells and basophils causing cell degranulation and release of mediators such as histamine, prostaglandins, leukotrienes and cytokines. These cause the symptoms and signs of anaphylaxis such as tachycardia, hypotension, bronchospasm, flushing and a rash.

2. What drugs are used in the treatment of anaphylaxis?
It is important to know the below drug doses off by heart as in an event of emergency. However do try and check if the situation permits.

AGE RANGE	ADRENALINE DOSE (MICROGRAMS)	VOLUME OF ADRENALINE 1 IN 1000 (1 MG/ML)
Under 6 years	150	0.15 ml
6 – 12 years	300	0.3 ml
12 – 18 years	500	0.5 ml

Doses of adrenaline can be repeated at 5 minute intervals depending on the patient's vital signs.

AGE RANGE	CHLORPHENAMINE	HYDROCORTISONE
Under 6 months	250 micrograms	25 mg
6 months – 6 years	2.5 mg	50 mg
6 – 12 years	5 mg	100 mg
12 – 18 years	10 mg	200 mg

Case 2 – **Testicular Torsion**

You are the FY2 doctor working in the Children's Emergency Department. You have been asked to see a 12-year-old boy, Jack Stone. He is complaining of severe abdominal and left sided scrotal pain that came on suddenly. He is also nauseous and has vomited twice.

Please conduct an A to E assessment of Jack Stone and commence the initial management.

Latest observations:
HR: 115 BP: 112/70 RR: 17 SaO_2 99 % (RA) Temp 37.2 °C UO: NA

Danger

It is safe to approach the patient

Response

Patient is talking to you

Airway

Airway is patent

Breathing

Normal respiratory assessment

Circulation

Normal cardiovascular assessment

Disability

AVPU – alert/GCS15
Blood glucose – 4.9
Pupils – equal and reactive to light

Exposure

You notice that Jack's left testicle is red, swollen and tender to touch. It is high riding and has a transverse lie. The pain is not alleviated by elevating the scrotum. There is also no cremasteric reflex on the left side. The abdomen is soft and non-tender.

At this stage you should suspect testicular torsion which is a urological emergency. Intra-venous access should be obtained and a set of pre-operative bloods (FBC,U&E clotting, Group and Save) should be taken.

This patient should be offered pain relief and anti-emetics (morphine and ondansetron) and have a urinary catheter inserted. He should then immediately be referred to the urology team for an operation to attempt testicular salvage. An ultrasound scan of the scrotum can be ordered to confirm the diagnosis, however this should not delay the surgery.

Hand over patient to Mr Grey (Urology SpR)

Situation – Hello Mr Grey, this is _____, the FY2 in A&E. I am calling you regarding Jack Stone, a 12 year old boy, who I suspect has testicular torsion.

Background – He presented to A&E with sudden onset left sided testicular pain associated with nausea and vomiting as well as abdominal pain.

Assessment – He has a tachycardia of 115 bpm, but otherwise his general examination is unremarkable. He has a red, swollen, tender, high riding left testicle with a horizontal lie. The pain is not diminished by elevating the scrotum and cremasteric reflex is absent on the affected side.

His last meal was 8 hours ago and I have made him nil by mouth and gave IV morphine and ondansetron to alleviate the pain and nausea. I also sent off bloods, requested a doppler ultrasound scan and inserted a urinary catheter. I will call theatres to make them aware that we have a potential case.

Recommendation – I would appreciate if you could come and review Jack. In the meantime, is there anything else you would like me to do?

Testicular torsion in brief

1. What is testicular torsion?

Testicular torsion is a urological emergency. It occurs when the spermatic cord twists on itself and the blood supply to the testicle is cut off, resulting in ischaemia. The commonest cause is a congenital malformation known as bell-clapper deformity, when the testis is not fixed to the scrotum and is more prone to twisting.

The diagnosis can be made clinically and it is imperative that the treatment is initiated as quickly as possible because irreversible ischaemia sets in approximately six hours after onset and could lead to the loss of the testicle.

It is important that children with undescended testes are referred for repair to reduce their risk of developing testicular torsion and testicular cancer in the future.

2. How is testicular torsion managed?

It is important to have immediate surgical input in such cases in order to save the testicle. Patients should be given pain relief and anti emetics. Detorsion with an orchidectomy or an orchidopexy should be performed as soon as possible. As a general rule the contralateral testicle is fixed during the same operation as it is also at an increased risk of torsion.

Manual de-torsion can be attempted if surgery is not available within the next six hours.

It is important to consider the psychological impact of an orchidectomy. Prosthetic devices can be offered to these patients.

Case 3 – **Acute Appendicitis**

You are a Foundation Year 2 doctor working in the Emergency Department. A 13-year-old boy, Adam Smith, has been brought in by his parents complaining of abdominal pain and vomiting.

Please conduct an A to E assessment of Adam Smith and commence the initial management.

Latest observations:
HR: 120 BP: 110/75 RR: 18 SaO$_2$: 100 % (RA) Temp: 37.5 °C UO: NA

Danger
It is safe to approach the patient.

Response
The patient is alert.

Airway
He tells you that his "tummy hurts" and it started 3 days ago. He vomited once this morning and hasn't had any appetite the past few days. It is safe to assume airway is patent.

Breathing
Look – no respiratory distress
Feel – trachea is central, chest expansion is symmetrical, percussion note is resonant
Listen – vesicular breath sounds throughout, no added sounds
Measure – RR: 18 SaO_2: 100 % (RA)
Treat – move on

Circulation
Look – distressed, JVP not raised, no pallor, no sunken eyes, moist mucous membranes
Feel – sweaty, regular rapid pulse and normal skin turgor
Listen – normal heart sounds
Measure – HR: 120 BP: 110/75 Temp: 37.5 °C CRT 2 s UO: NA
Treat – obtain IV access, commence fluid replacement therapy (based on daily requirements and urine output), monitor fluid balance and give paracetamol for pain and pyrexia.
Reassess – HR: 95 BP: 120/82 Temp: 37.0 °C, CRT 2 s.

Further investigations:
- Bloods (FBC, U&E, LFT, CRP, clotting screen, amylase)
- Dipstick urine sample

Disability

AVPU – Alert/GCS 15
Blood glucose – 4.5 mmol/L
Pupils – Equal and reactive to light

Exposure

Fully expose the patient and perform an abdominal examination. On examination there is no distension, the abdomen is very tender in the right iliac fossa (RIF) and there is guarding but no masses palpable. Rovsing's sign positive (RIF pain with palpation of left iliac fossa). Bowel sounds are present. Keep patient nil by mouth.

Hand over to Mr Steward (Surgical SpR)

Situation – Hello Mr Steward, my name is _____ and I am the FY2 in A&E. I am calling about a 13-year-old boy, Adam Smith, with acute appendicitis.

Background – He came in with a 3-day history of abdominal pain, anorexia and he vomited once this morning.

Assessment – On initial assessment, he was tachycardic HR 120 with a temperature of 37.5 °C but other parameters were normal. On examination of his abdomen, there was guarding and he was very tender in the right iliac fossa and Rovsing's positive. No masses were felt. I have inserted two cannulae, taken bloods and ordered an abdominal ultrasound. I have also kept him nil by mouth and given him maintenance fluids and paracetamol. His urine dipstick was negative.

Recommendation – I would like you to come and review this patient and consider taking him to theatre. Is there anything else you would like me to do in the meantime?

Acute appendicitis in brief

1. What scoring system can be used to help determine the need for further investigation and treatment in suspected acute appendicitis?

The Alvarado scoring system

FEATURE	SCORE
Migratory RIF pain	1
Anorexia	1
Nausea or vomiting	1
Tenderness in RIF	2
Rebound tenderness in RIF	1
Elevated temperature	1
Leucocytosis	2
Left shift of neutrophils	1
Total	10

From a total possible score of 10, further investigation with a CT scan has been recommended for scores 4-6, and consideration of appendicectomy for scores of 7 and above.

2. What are the complications of acute appendicitis?

1. **Perforation** – Commoner if faecolith is present and in young children due to delayed diagnosis. The average rate of perforation at presentation is between 16 and 30 %.

2. **Appendix mass** – Caused by omentum and small bowel adhering to the inflamed appendix. Usually presents with a fever and palpable mass. Initial management is conservative with fluids, analgesia and antibiotics. Surgical intervention is required if the mass enlarges or the patient deteriorates.

3. **Appendix abscess** – May occur if an appendix mass fails to resolve but enlarges and the patient becomes more unwell. Can be demonstrated on ultrasound or CT scan. Conservative treatment with antibiotics alone may be sufficient or the patient can be treated with percutaneous or open drainage.

Case 4 – **Non-Accidental Injury**

You are a Foundation Year 2 doctor working the night shift in the Emergency Department. A 6-year-old boy, Eric Taylor, presents with abdominal pain and pain in his left arm. His mother, Mrs Taylor, has brought him in just now even though she tells you that he fell off the swing the previous morning.

Please conduct an A to E assessment of Eric and commence the initial management

Latest observations:

HR 100; BP 110/90; RR 15; SpO$_2$ 100 % (on room air); temp 37.1 °C UO: not available

Danger
It is safe to approach Eric.

Response
Eric is shy and talks minimally. He does not make eye contact with you.

Airway
Eric is able to talk (airway is patent).

Breathing
Normal respiratory examination.

Circulation
Normal cardiovascular examination.

Disability
AVPU – alert/GCS 15
Capillary blood glucose – 5.9 mmol/L
Pupils – equal and reactive to light. Normal neurological examination

Exposure
Eric appears to be cradling his left arm.
On examination:
- Abdominal examination – soft abdomen, there is some bruising over the left upper quadrant and the area is tender to touch.
- Musculo-skeletal examination - refusing to move the left arm due to pain. Does not want you to touch his left arm as it's very painful. The gait and the range of motion in all other limbs are normal.

On further exposure you note:
- Multiple linear bruises on his buttocks,
- Multiple circular scars on his back, along with a fresh small circular burn on his left shoulder
- You also note a well-circumscribed first degree burn of his left ankle in a sock pattern.

Further investigations
- Upper limb X-ray - spiral fracture of the left radius and ulna.

Ensure to document everything accurately in the notes, as this may be used later in court as evidence.

Handover the patient to Dr Lister (Paediatrics SpR)

Situation – Good evening Dr Lister my name is _____ and I am the F2 in A&E. I am calling regarding Eric Taylor, a 6-year-old boy. I am concerned regarding non-accidental injury as this boy has presented with suspicious injuries.

Background – He was brought in by his mother with a delayed presentation following a fall from a swing yesterday morning.

Assessment – He appears shy and withdrawn with poor eye contact and ability to communicate. He has numerous fresh linear bruises on his buttocks and suspicious circular scars and burns on his back and left ankle. An upper limb x-ray reveals a spiral fracture of his left radius and ulna, which are inconsistent with the history of his fall.

Recommendation – I would like you to come and review him, as I feel that these are suspicious circumstances, which suggest non-accidental injury. Is there anything you would like me to do until you are able to attend?

Non-accidental injury (NAI) in brief

1. What features in a history would be suggestive of a NAI?
History of presenting complaint:
- Inconsistent or self-inflicted injury - history of the mechanism of injury constantly changes, or injuries are reported to be caused by the child
- Vague or unexplained mechanism of injury
- A delay in presentation to the hospital
- Repeated hospital presentations or frequent injuries
- Injuries inconsistent with the developmental capacity of the child
- Injuries that occur between midnight and 6am.

General history:
- Global developmental delay
- Poor weight and height gain
- Poor school performance
- Behavioural issues
- Inconsistent vaccination history

2. **What physical examination findings are suggestive of a NAI?**
a) Bruises that
    i) Resemble various objects
    ii) Appear in clusters
    iii) Are of constant shape or size

b) Location of bruises in unusual places:
    i) Non-bony areas
    ii) Face, eyes, ears
    iii) Neck and top of the shoulder
    iv) Inner arms
    v) Anterior chest
    vi) Abdomen
    vii) Groins and the inner thigh

c) Burns that
    i) Are multiple
    ii) Have a clearly demarcated edge
    iii) In unusual areas: back, shoulders, dorsum of the hands, soles of feet and buttocks

3. **What should you do if you suspect a NAI?**
a) Take a complete history in a non-judgmental or accusatory manner
b) Clearly document the history and all the physical findings (can be used in court at a later date)
c) Document the reasons for your suspicion
d) Notify your senior colleague and social services
e) Do not discharge the patient if you suspect that they are at risk

Case 5 – **Acute Exacerbation of Asthma in a Child**

You are a Foundation Year 2 doctor working in the Emergency Department. A 5-year-old boy, Tariq Mizra, presents with tightness in his chest and increasing shortness of breath. An audible wheeze is also heard. He has a past medical history of asthma and was last hospitalised with an acute exacerbation three months ago.

Please conduct an A to E assessment of Tariq and commence the initial management.

Latest observations:

HR 140; BP 95/50; RR 45; SpO$_2$ 90 % (on room air); temp 36.5 °C UO: not available

Danger
It is safe to approach Tariq

Response
Tariq is drowsy, and responds in short single words

Airway
Look – no signs of airway obstruction or evidence of oedema
Feel – it is clear that he is breathing so no need to feel for movement of air
Listen – audible wheeze is heard from the end of the bed
Treat – adjust his position so that he is sitting upright

Breathing
Look – agitated, no cyanosis, using accessory muscles; he is unable to complete full sentences, but is able to answer in single words
Feel – the trachea is central; minimal chest expansion
Listen – on auscultation there is minimal air entry and bilateral wheeze
Measure – RR 45; SpO_2 90 % (on room air)
Treat – give high-flow oxygen via a non-rebreathe mask to maintain SaO_2 between 94 – 98 %. Give burst therapy (single dose of steroids: prednisolone orally or intravenous hydrocortisone (if vomiting)); three back to back doses of nebulised salbutamol and ipratropium.
Reassess – his saturations rise to 99 % on 15 L of oxygen and RR is now 30. He appears to be slightly more comfortable and less agitated. The air entry has slightly improved, however the wheeze persists

Since the patient failed to adequately respond to the initial treatment, he should continue receiving back-to-back salbutamol nebulisers and escalation of treatment to paediatric high dependency unit (HDU) should be considered.

Further investigations:
- Attempt to measure Peak Expiratory Flow Rate (PEFR). However, this may be difficult in a child this old.
- Consider a chest x-ray (if first presentation).

Circulation

Look – appears pale and clammy, central cyanosis
Feel – apex beat is not displaced, warm peripheries, normal skin turgor
Listen – normal heart sounds, with no added heart sounds
Measure – HR 140 bpm, regular; BP 95/5; CRT <2 seconds; UO: not available; temp 36.5 °C
Treat – obtain IV access and consider further investigations

> If the patient fails to respond to the treatment with steroids, salbutamol and ipratropium, you should consider starting aminophylline and magnesium sulphate following a discussion with your seniors.

Further investigations:
- ECG monitoring and continuous monitoring of BP (if considering magnesium sulphate treatment)
- Bloods (FBC, U&E – if aminophylline considered, Mg^{2+} levels – if considering magnesium sulphate)

Disability

AVPU – alert/GCS 13(E3, V4, M6)
Capillary blood glucose – 5.9 mmol/L
Pupils/neurology – equal and reactive to light; moving all 4 limbs

Exposure

Fully expose the patient and perform a detailed secondary examination – nothing of note.

Hand over the patient to Dr Lister (Paediatric SpR)

Situation – Good morning Dr Lister my name is _____ and I am the F2 in A&E. I am calling regarding Tariq Mizra, a 5 year old boy who has presented with an acute life-threatening exacerbation of asthma.

Background – He is a known asthmatic with previous hospital admissions the last one being three months ago.

Assessment – He improved after the administration of nebulised salbutamol, ipratropium and oral steroids but I am worried that he remains unstable. His airway is clear. His respiratory rate has improved from 45 to 28; his saturations are 99 % on 15 L and after burst therapy. His HR, BP, and CRT are all within normal limits and he is apyrexial. He is drowsy at present and his blood capillary glucose was 5.9 mmol/L.

Recommendation – I would like for you to come and review him, as he remains tachypnoeic and I feel he may need to go to HDU (High Dependency Unit) for close monitoring and treatment with magnesium sulphate and aminophylline. I have obtained IV access. Is there anything else you would like to me to do until you are able to attend?

Paediatric asthma in brief

1. What are the normal paediatric observation parameters?

AGE	RESPIRATORY RATE		HEART RATE		SYSTOLIC BP	
	Max	Min	Max	Min	Max	Min
<1 y/o	40	30	160	110	90	70
2 – 5 y/o	30	20	140	90	100	80
5 – 12 y/o	20	15	120	80	110	90
>12 y/o	16	12	100	60	120	100

NB
- Estimation of minimum systolic BP = 70 + (2 x Age in years)
- Estimation of weight = (2 x Age in years) + 7

2. How do you assess the severity of paediatric asthma?

Assessment of severity and the subsequent management of asthma in the paediatric population is spilt into two age groups, the 2 – 5 year-olds and those greater than 5. Children below the age of 2 are unlikely to have asthma and an alternative diagnosis should be considered. Those above the age of 12 should be treated in the same way as adults.

AGE	MODERATE	SEVERE	LIFE-THREATENING
2 – 5 y/o	• SpO_2 ≥92 %	• SpO_2 <92 % • Too breathless to eat/talk • Use of accessory muscles • HR >140 bpm • RR >40 /min	• SpO_2 <92 % • Silent chest • Poor respiratory effort • Agitation/altered consciousness • Cyanosis
>5 y/o	• SpO_2 ≥92 % • PEFR >50 %	• SpO_2 <92 % • PEFR = 33 to 50 % • Unable to complete full sentences • Use of accessory muscles • HR >125 bpm • RR >30/min	• SpO_2 ≤92 % • PEFR <33 % • Silent chest • Poor respiratory effort • Agitation/altered consciousness • Cyanosis

3. What further treatments should be considered if the patient remains unresponsive to initial burst therapy?

- Repeat nebulised salbutamol and nebulised ipratropium bromide
- IV salbutamol bolus or consider continuous IV salbutamol infusion. This will require continuous cardiac monitoring.
- Consider IV aminophylline or IV magnesium sulphate (if >5 years old)
    → IV aminophylline loading dose followed by an IV aminopylline infusion
    → IV magnesium sulphate infusion
- If giving magnesium sulphate continuous cardiac monitoring will be required
- If giving aminophylline perform baseline U&Es

Case 6 – **Paediatric Basic Life Support**

You are a Foundation Year 1 doctor working on a busy paediatric ward. You have just finished your shift and are about to leave when you notice one of your patients in the side room. It's a five-year-old boy, James Rowen, who was admitted with a severe bout of food poisoning. You notice he is slumped over. There is a tray of food in front of him.

Please conduct an A-E assessment of James Rowen and commence the initial management.

Latest observations:
Unavailable

Danger
It is safe to approach the patient.

Response
Patient is unresponsive.

Airway
Look – a piece of food lodged at the back of the throat, the chest is not rising
Feel – no breaths or pulse felt
Listen – no breath sounds

Call for help or press the emergency buzzer

Treat – remove the foreign body using Magill forceps. Perform a head-tilt-chin-lift. Commence 5 rescue breaths. If oxygen available, start 15 L/min via non-rebreathe mask.
Reassess – no signs of life

Commence the paediatric BLS algorithm and ask for the paediatric crash team to be called.

Continue cycle of 2 rescue breaths and 15 chest compressions until help arrives.

Paediatric basic life support in brief

Paediatric BLS chart (Adapted from Resuscitation Council UK)

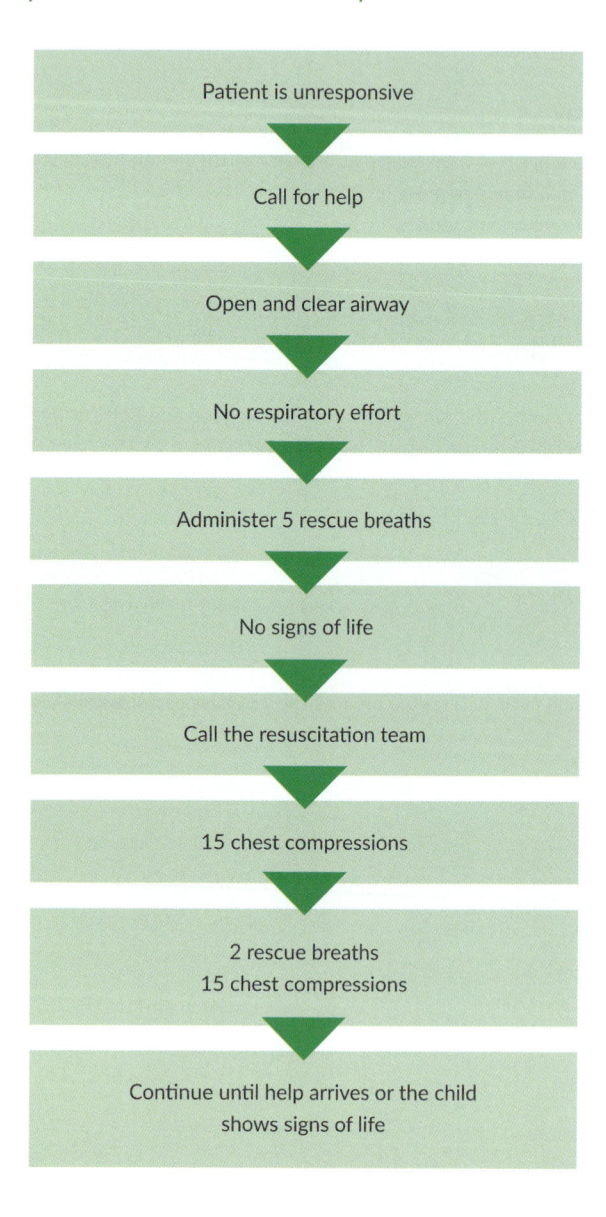

- Patient is unresponsive
- Call for help
- Open and clear airway
- No respiratory effort
- Administer 5 rescue breaths
- No signs of life
- Call the resuscitation team
- 15 chest compressions
- 2 rescue breaths
  15 chest compressions
- Continue until help arrives or the child shows signs of life

1. How is paediatric life support different from adult BLS?

Never perform a blind finger sweep in children. Their palates are very susceptible to damage.

Head-tilt-chin-lift should not be performed in infants (age <1). Their head should be kept in the neutral position, when starting CPR.

Breathing and circulation should be assessed within 10 seconds. If unsure, treat it as abnormal and commence CPR.

Assess circulation by palpating the brachial or femoral pulses.

If the child starts breathing again but remains unconscious, place them in the recovery position.

Chest compressions:

In children up to 6 years of age rest your thumbs side by side on the lower part of the sternum. Your thumbs should wrap around the lower ribcage and support the back. Press down on the sternum to a 1/3 of the depth of the child's chest.

In children older than 6, compressions are performed in the same manner as in adults, however initially with only one hand and with adjusted force.

Chest compressions should be performed at a rate of 100 – 120 per minute.

CPR should continue until:
- The child begins showing signs of life, either by coughing, moving or if their pulse is greater than 60 bpm
- Help arrives
- You have become exhausted

2. What are the common causes of cardiopulmonary arrest in children?

Hypoxia and hypovolaemia are usually the underlying cause of cardiopulmonary arrest in children. Common underlying causes include::
- Respiratory conditions, like asthma and bronchiolitis
- Anaphylaxis
- Sepsis
- Trauma
- Drug overdose

Case 7 – **Upper Airway Obstruction**

You are a Foundation Year 2 doctor working in the Emergency Department. A 2-year-old girl, Anna Bailey, presents with a worsening cough and struggling to breathe. Symptoms have worsened over the past 3 hours. Her mother, Mrs Maureen Bailey is present. She reports that Anna has been feeling unwell and lethargic over the past 2 days.

Please conduct an A to E assessment of Anna and commence the initial management.

Latest observations:

HR 150; BP 100/80; RR 35; SpO$_2$ 92 % (on room air); temp 37.5 °C; UO: not available

Danger

It is safe to approach Anna

Response

Anna is alert and responsive. She is coughing and has a hoarse voice.

Airway

Look – no signs of upper airway obstruction
Feel – do not feel in order not to agitate the child
Listen – a loud, high-pitched inspiratory noise is heard (stridor) and a barking cough is noted
Treat – adjust her position so that she is sitting upright

Breathing

Look – alert, mild perioral cyanosis noted; mild chest wall retractions
Feel – no need to feel the trachea (in order to avoid agitating the child)
Listen – stridor noted, decreased air entry bilaterally
Measure – RR 35; SpO_2 92 % (on room air)
Treat – give high-flow oxygen via a non-rebreathe mask to maintain SpO_2 between 94 – 98 %. Give nebulised 1:1000 adrenaline. Give oral dexamethasone if able to swallow OR nebulised budesonide.
Reassess – her saturations rise to 98 % on 10 L of oxygen and RR is now 30.

Further investigations:
- Chest x-ray to exclude foreign body obstruction or tapering of the upper trachea (suggestive of croup)

Circulation

Look – pale, no cyanosis
Feel – apex beat is not displaced, warm peripheries, normal skin turgor
Listen – normal heart sounds
Measure - HR 150 bpm and regular; BP 100/80; CRT <2 seconds; temp 37.5 °C; UO: not available
Treat – monitor heart rate

Disability

AVPU – alert/GCS 15
Capillary blood glucose – 5.9 mmol/L
Pupils/neurology – equal and reactive to light, moving all four limbs

Exposure

Fully expose the patient and perform a detailed secondary examination – nothing of note.

Hand over the patient to Dr Lister (Paediatric SpR)

Situation – Good morning Dr Lister my name is _____ and I am the F2 in A&E. I am calling regarding Anna Bailey, a 2 year old girl. The reason I am calling is that I am concerned she may have severe croup.

Background – She has presented with a barking cough and stridor over the last 3 hours. She has also been feeling unwell and lethargic over the past 2 days.

Assessment – She has improved after administration of nebulised adrenaline and oral dexamethasone, but I am worried that she remains unstable. Her airway is clear at present. Her respiratory rate has improved from 35 to 30; her saturations are currently 98 % on 10 L of oxygen. Her HR, BP, and CRT are all within normal limits and she is apyrexial. She is alert at present and her blood capillary glucose was 5.9 mmol/L.

Recommendation – I would like for you to come and review her, as she remains on high flow oxygen and I feel she may need to go to HDU for close monitoring. I have scheduled a chest X-ray to exclude a foreign body inhalation. Is there anything you would like me to do until you are able to attend?

Upper airway obstruction causes in brief

1. What are the differentials to consider when a child presents with stridor?

FOREIGN BODY INHALATION	CROUP	BACTERIAL TRACHEITIS	EPIGLOTTITIS
Common	Common	Uncommon	Rare
Any age	6 m/o – 6 y/o	6 m/o – 14 y/o	2 – 7 y/o
Sudden onset	Onset over a few days	Viral prodrome 2 – 5d, rapid ↓↓	Sudden onset
Cough / Choking	Harsh Stridor when upset	Continuous Biphasic Stridor	Soft Continuous Stridor
			Drooling of secretions
Hoarse voice	Hoarse voice	Very hoarse voice	Soft voice
Apyrexial	Apyrexial, barking cough	Moderate-high fever, barking cough	Toxic + feverish, no cough

2. What is croup?

Croup, also known as laryngotracheobronchitis, is a common childhood acute viral infection of the upper airways. The symptoms of croup result from inflammation and obstruction of the upper airways. The parainfluenza virus is commonly responsible. Diphtheria can also cause a bacterial croup-like illness but is now rare in the western world because of a widespread vaccination programme.

3. How would you assess the severity of croup?

Assessment of severity is mainly based on clinical findings, with signs of respiratory distress being the most important (amount of chest wall recession, cyanosis and agitation). Signs of impending respiratory failure are important to remember:
- Changes in mental state or consciousness
- Pallor
- Tachycardia (a late sign)

A commonly used scoring system is the Westley croup score, which is based on some of these symptoms (chest wall reactions, stridor, cyanosis, air entry and level of consciousness).
- <2 – mild disease
- 3 – 7 – moderate disease
- >7 severe disease

4. What are the important things to consider in the management of upper airway obstruction?

Early correct diagnosis of the cause of the upper airway obstruction is important, since the management of these diseases varies greatly. However, it is important to ensure that the child is not further agitated by any interventions or actions as in all cases the obstruction may worsen. Often it is helpful to involve the parents in helping to keep the child calm. For example, allow them to put on the oxygen mask.

In croup, the mainstay of treatment is early administration of glucocorticoids. In mild croup, oral dexamethasone and supplementary oxygen are often sufficient. Nebulised adrenaline is used in more severe cases as an adjunct to the steroids and provides symptomatic relief.

If the above measures fail, and the child is becoming progressively hypoxic and hypercarbic, intubation will be required.

Psychiatric Emergencies
Estelle Yeak

Acute Alcohol Withdrawal	322
Delirium	326
Neuroleptic Malignant Syndrome	332
Wernicke's Encephalopathy	334

Case 1 – **Acute Alcohol Withdrawal**

You are a Foundation Year 1 doctor covering the acute medical unit (AMU) at night. One of the AMU nurses rushes into the office and tells you that Mr. Tremayne, a 49-year-old man, just had a fit. You are aware from the hand over that Mr. Tremayne was admitted 48 hours ago for IV antibiotic treatment of his right leg cellulitis. You also note from the hand over sheet that Mr. Tremayne has a significant history of excessive alcohol consumption. The nurse tells you that he has been quiet, anxious, irritable and shaky in the evening. Since then he wasn't able to fall asleep and appeared confused, complaining of ants in his bed.

Please conduct an A to E assessment of Mr. Tremayne and commence the initial management.

Latest observations:
HR: 138 BP: 157/99 RR: 24 SaO$_2$: 98 % (RA) Temp: 37.0 °C UO: NA

Danger

The patient is agitated.

You should take care when approaching and assessing an agitated patient and it is recommended for another person to accompany you.

Response

The patient is confused and cannot answer your questions coherently

Airway

Look – there is some vomit around the mouth
Feel – some vomit in the mouth (wear gloves)
Listen – some gurgling sounds
Treat – recognise an airway at risk, ask for a Yankauer suction tip and clear it
Reassess – airway is now patent, move on

Breathing

Look – the patient is tachypnoeaic, no central cyanosis or accessory muscle use
Feel – normal tracheal position, chest expansion and percussion note
Listen – normal breath sounds bilaterally
Measure – RR 24, SaO_2 98 % (on room air)
Treat – move on

Circulation

Look – the patient appears sweaty and pale
Feel – warm to touch, CRT <2 s
Listen – normal heart sounds
Measure - HR: 138 BP: 157/99 Temp: 37.0 °C UO: NA
Treat – it is important to ensure that this patient has a patent cannula in situ since he will require IV treatment
Reassess – move on

Disability

AVPU – responds to voice/GCS 11 (E3V3M5)
Blood glucose – 4.9 mmol/L
Pupils – equal and reactive to light

Exposure

Whilst exposing the patient he starts to fit again. What will you do now?

1. Assess and secure the airway
2. Administer oxygen via a facemask (5 – 10 L)
3. Give IV benzodiazepines (lorazepam or diazepam)

At this point it would be appropriate to call for senior help as this patient may require ITU admission. If seizures continue, treat it as status epilepticus (see the Status Epilepticus case). Once the seizures stop it is important to reassess the patient using the A-E approach, take a history and perform a detailed secondary examination.

Hand over the patient to Dr Conway (Acute Medicine SpR)

Situation – This is Dr_____, the night FY1 on AMU. I have just seen Mr Tremayne, a 49-year-old man with seizures, which I suspect are due to acute alcohol withdrawal.

Background – Mr. Tremayne was admitted 48 hours ago for IV antibiotic treatment of right leg cellulitis. He has a history of excessive alcohol consumption. The nurse also reports that the patient has recently been feeling anxious, irritable and shaky. He was also confused and was hallucinating.

Assessment – On initial assessment the patient appeared drowsy and confused and could not converse coherently. His airway was initially compromised with some vomit but this resolved following suction. The patient was tachypnoeaic, but had bilateral normal air entry and was saturating well on room air. The patient was also tachycardic at 138 bpm and hypertensive at 157/99. He was responsive to voice and his GCS was 12. During the examination the patient started fitting and I gave him intravenous lorazepam, which terminated the seizures.

Recommendation – I suspect this patient is suffering from delirium tremens. I would like you to review this patient as soon as possible. Would you like me to initiate treatment for acute alcohol withdrawal in the meantime?

> **Box 1.** **Management of acute alcohol withdrawal**
>
> Benzodiazepines are considered to be the first line for alcohol related seizures and withdrawal symptoms. Drugs such as lorazepam, diazepam or chlordiazepoxide may be used. Patients may require vitamin supplementation. Thiamine should be given before carbohydrates if the patient is at risk of developing Wernicke's encephalopathy. Folic acid and magnesium should also be considered.

Acute alcohol withdrawal in brief:

1. What is the pathophysiology of acute alcohol withdrawal?
It is thought that alcohol reduces the concentration of glutamate in the brain, which leads to an increase in NMDA receptors. When alcohol is abruptly stopped, there is loss of glutamate inhibition and brain over-excitation occurs. Alcohol has also been shown to reduce the activity of GABA, the main inhibitory neurotransmitter in the brain.

2. What is the mechanism of action of benzodiazepines?
Benzodiazepines modulate the activity of the GABA receptor in the brain increasing presynaptic inhibition.

3. What is the difference between Wernicke's encephalopathy and Korsakoff syndrome?
Wernicke-Korsakoff syndrome is a spectrum of neurological and higher cognitive dysfunction as a result of thiamine (vitamin B_1) deficiency, commonly encountered in alcoholics. Wernicke's encephalopathy is characterised by a triad of: ataxia, ophthalmoplegia and confusion. Korsakoff syndrome lies on the far end of the spectrum and is characterised by anterograde and retrograde amnesia with lack of insight and confabulation.

Case 2 – **Delirium**

You are a geriatrics Foundation Year 1 doctor. A nurse has bleeped you from the care of the elderly ward. Over the phone she says that Mr Thomas Blakemore, a 90 year old gentleman, has begun walking up and down the ward shouting, accusing the nurses of being devils from hell and attempting to go home. He was admitted yesterday for a urinary tract infection due to his benign prostatic hyperplasia. She would like you to come and assess the patient.

Please conduct an A to E assessment of Mr. Blakemore and commence the initial management.

Latest observations:
HR: 90 BP: 120/80 RR: 21 SaO$_2$: 97 % (RA) Temp: 38.5 °C UO: 14 mls in the last hour

Danger

He is really agitated and shouting loudly.

Your safety is important and you should therefore assess the patient with a colleague

Response

The patient looks at you belligerently. "You are the devil," he says.

You should keep calm, maintain eye contact and an open body posture. Introduce yourself. Suggest that you go to a quiet room to talk. Try to negotiate with the patient that you need to assess him. The patient is more likely to be compliant as long as you remain calm. Take care to maintain good communication skills throughout the rest of the assessment. If the patient fails to settle, hospital security should be called.

Airway

Patient is talking. You can assume the airway is patent

Breathing

Look – not cyanosed
Feel – equal chest expansion, resonant percussion
Listen – vesicular breathing, no added sounds
Measure – RR 21, SaO_2: 97 % (on room air)
Treat – continuously monitor SaO_2 for deterioration. Move on

Circulation

Look – flushed, red
Feel – warm, sweaty palms, apex beat not displaced
Listen – normal heart sounds
Measure – HR: 104, BP 120/80, CRT 2 s Temp: 38.5 °C UO: 14mls in the last hour (catheterised)
Treat – inspect the catheter bag, and flush the catheter to ensure it is working. Prescribe maintenance fluids and paracetamol.
Reassess – move on

Further investigations:
- Bloods (FBC, U&E, CRP)
- Blood cultures
- Urine dipstick and send off a sample for microbiology and culture
- ECG – demonstrates sinus tachycardia

Disability

AVPU – Patient is alert/GCS14 (E4V4M6)
Blood glucose – 5.5 mmol/L
Pupils – Equal and reactive to light

You should also perform the Abbreviated Mental Test Score (AMTS) (see Delirium in brief)

Exposure

On further examination you feel a large tender mass in the suprapubic region, which extends to the umbilicus. It is dull to percussion and you are able to get above it. You should perform an ultrasound examination of the bladder at this stage. This shows a distended bladder with 900 mL.

You should therefore attempt to flush this patient's catheter and if this fails you should change the catheter, which should then drain approximately 900 mL of urine. The patient settles following the catheter change.

In patients who present with delirium the underlying cause should be treated first. If this fails other measures can be attempted (see Box 1.)

Hand over the patient to Dr Shah (Geriatrics SpR)

Situation – Hello my name is _____, and I am the geriatrics FY1 doctor on call. I am calling regarding Mr Thomas Blakemore a 90 year old gentleman who is extremely agitated on the ward and I suspect is delirious.

Background – He was admitted for urinary tract infection and obstruction, with a past medical history of benign prostatic hyperplasia.

Assessment – Before assessing him I have moved him to a quiet room in order to de-escalate the situation. His respiratory examination was normal but he was tachycardic at 104 bpm with a normal blood pressure. He had a low urinary output and he was pyrexic with a temperature of 38.5 °C. He had a distended bladder with 900 mL of urine. I believe this gentleman was suffering from delirium, secondary to a catheter obstruction and possibly a urinary tract infection. His urine dipstick had 3+ protein, nitrates and leucocytes and I therefore sent off urinary cultures to the lab to confirm this.

Recommendation – I have flushed the catheter which then drained 900 mL of urine and the patient has settled down. I have also given the patient 1 g of paracetamol for the fever. I was wondering if we should start him on antibiotics and if there is anything else you would like me to do?

Box 1. Management of agitated patients:

In order to de-escalate the situation, one individual should take over the role of communicating with the patient. Taking the patient into a quiet room will aid with the de-escalation. However it is important not to stay with the patient on your own as they may become violent. You should use communication techniques such as body language and eye contact to calm the patient down.

The underlying cause of the delirium should then be treated and this will resolve the delirium in most cases. If this fails and the patient is starting to become a danger to himself or those around him, consider medication. However, do discuss the patient with your seniors prior to this. The medicines that can be used include:
- Haloperidol (contraindicated in delirium tremens, Parkinson's disease or Lewy body dementia)
- Lorazepam

If medical treatment fails and the patient is still at risk to themselves or others restrictive measures should be considered. In these complex situations you should always consider what is in the patient's best interests. When restricting the patient you should employ the least restrictive intervention.

Delirium in brief

1. How do you differentiate delirium from psychosis?

Both delirium and psychosis can present similarly and result in increased mortality and morbidity among hospitalised patients. Delirium, also known as acute confusional state, usually presents with an altered level of consciousness, a change in mental status, disorganised thinking and inattention. Even though the aetiology of delirium is multifactorial, it is thought to be an organic disorder. It usually occurs in vunerable/frail individuals (ie. geriatric patients) with a reduced cognitive functional reserve, triggered by physiological insults such as infection, metabolic and electrolyte derangements, surgery, pain or medications.

Acute psychosis on the other hand results from abnormal dopaminergic transmission in frontal and temporal lobes. These patients usually present with disorganised thinking, hallucinations and delusions as well as personality changes. The cause of psychosis can be divided into primary and secondary. Primary causes include psychiatric disorders such as schizophrenia and schizoaffective disorder. Secondary causes of psychosis include psychotropic drugs such alcohol, cocaine and cannabis or medical disorders such as thiamine deficiency leading to Korsakoff's psychosis and acute porphyria.

One should suspect delirium over psychosis in an elderly patient with a fluctuating consciousness level.

2. What is the Abbreviated Mental Test Score (AMTS)

The AMTS is used to quickly assess the level of cognitive functioning particularly in the elderly patient. It is a good quick screening test to identify confusion or cognitive impairment, which would then require a further more detailed assessment.

The test consists of 10 questions:
1. Patient's age
2. Patient's date of birth
3. Current year
4. Time to the nearest hour
5. Name of the hospital
6. Current prime minister or monarch (or another well-known public figure)
7. Dates of World War 1 or 2 (or another well-known event)
8. Ability to recognise two people (ie. doctor and nurse)
9. Recalling the address: 42 West Registry Street
10. Counting backwards from 20 to 1

A score of <8 is abnormal and should prompt further investigations.

3. What are the causes of delirium?

There are multiple causes of delirium. Due to the high mortality and morbidity of the condition, each patient presenting with delirium should be fully investigated to avoid missing an important diagnosis.

The common causes are:
- Infection - by far the most common cause, and includes: urinary tract infections, respiratory infections and sepsis. Every patient with delirium should have a blood culture done.
- Pain – another common cause, particularly in ITU patients.
- Toxins and drugs - delirium can be secondary to consumption of various substances including alcohol, amphetamines, tricyclic antidepressants, opiates and corticosteroids.
- Myocardial infarction – occasionally elderly patients present with delirium, as the only feature for an underlying myocardial ischaemia. Every patient with delirium should therefore have an ECG done.
- Neurological disorders – stroke, meningitis/encephalitis. All patients with delirium should have an AMTS done, along with a brief neurological assessment. If there are any positive findings, a CT head or MRI should be considered.
- Respiratory disorders – hypoxia or hypercarbia can frequently cause delirium.
- Metabolic derangements - most commonly due to thyroid, sodium, potassium or calcium abnormalities. These are all potentially serious and should be investigated and treated urgently. Hypoglycaemia and hyperglycaemia can also present with delirium.

A good mnemonic to remember is PINCH ME (Pain, INfection, Constipation, Hydration, Metabolic, OthErs)

Case 3 – **Neuroleptic Malignant Syndrome**

You are an FY1 doctor working in psychiatry. Mr Jellal Jain, a 40 year old gentleman who has recently been diagnosed with schizophrenia, was admitted to your ward earlier in the week and started on chlorpromazine yesterday. A nurse asks you to review Mr Jain because for the past 10 hours he has been drowsy and developed muscle rigidity, "strange movements" and fever.

Please conduct an A to E assessment of Mr. Jain and commence the initial management.

Latest observations:
HR: 120 BP: 160/110 RR: 30 SaO_2: 80 % (RA) Temp: 39.5 °C UO: NA

Danger
The patient is not agitated and it is safe to approach him.

Response
The patient is unresponsive. You should therefore call for help.

Airway
Look – no obvious foreign bodies but visible excessive secretions
Feel – breath is felt
Listen – gurgling sounds present
Treat – perform a head-tilt-chin-lift manoeuvre and use a Yankauer sucker to suction the excess secretions.
Reassess – the airway is now clear, move on.

Breathing
Look – pursed lip breathing, central cyanosis
Feel – equal chest expansion, no tracheal deviation, percussion note is resonant
Listen – quiet breath sounds bilaterally
Measure – RR 30, O_2 SaO_2 80 % (on room air)
Treat – 15 L oxygen via non-rebreathe bag valve mask
Reassess – RR 26, SaO_2 95 % (on 15 L O_2)

Further investigations:
- Perform an ABG and consider a chest x-ray

Circulation
Look – pallor, JVP not visible
Feel – warm, CRT <2 s, apex beat not displaced
Listen – normal heart sounds
Measure – HR: 130, BP: 110/50, Temp: 39.5 °C, UO: NA
Treat – Gain IV access, and commence fluids to keep patient well hydrated, give antipyretics (eg. paracetamol). Also consider cooled blankets, ice packs, cooled fluids
Reassess – HR: 110, BP 120/70, temp still 38.4 °C

Further investigations:
- Bloods (FBC, U&E, LFT, CRP, CK)
- Bloods cultures
- ECG (sinus tachycardia)

Disability

AVPU – patient responds to pain/GCS9 (E2V3M4)
Blood glucose – 5.5 mmol/L
Pupils – equal and reactive to light

Exposure

The patient's body is stiff and rigid. You note a small tremor in the hands. There are no rashes and the abdomen is soft and non-tender.

> You should suspect neuroleptic malignant syndrome at this stage, stop the chlorpromazine, and start a muscle relaxant (i.e. dantrolene sodium).

Hand over the patient to Dr Ramprakash (Critical Care SpR)

Situation – Good evening Dr Ramprakash, I am _____ , the psychiatry FY1. I am calling regarding Mr Jellal Jain a 40 year old gentleman who I suspect has neuroleptic malignant syndrome.

Background – Mr Jellal was recently diagnosed with schizophrenia and has been started on chlorpromazine yesterday. I have been asked to see him because he developed muscle rigidity, pyrexia and became drowsy.

Assessment – On assessment he was poorly responsive, with sialorrhoea. He was tachypnoeic and hypoxic 80 % on room air, tachycardic at 120 bpm, hyperthermic at 39.5 °C with a labile blood pressure ranging from an initial 160/80 to 110/50. I have cleared his airway, and initiated oxygen therapy with 15 L of oxygen through a non-rebreathe mask. His SaO_2 are now 95 % on 15 L O_2. I have started the patient on antipyretics and a cooled fluid challenge. His BP is now 120/65. I have also stopped his chlorpromazine and started him on dantrolene sodium.

Recommendation – I think this gentleman has had a reaction to his chlorpromazine. I would like you to come and assess him as soon as possible. Would you like me to do anything in the meantime?

Neuroleptic malignant syndrome in brief

1. What is the definition of neuroleptic malignant syndrome (NMS)
It is a rare but life threatening reaction to abrupt reduction in dopamine or dopamine agonist availability. It can occur as a result of neuroleptic antipsychotic medication administration or in Parkinson's disease when dopamine agonists are abruptly withdrawn.

It is characterized by muscle rigidity, hyperthermia, alterations in the autonomic nervous system and an altered mental state. It should be noted that these symptoms are also caused by other conditions such as sepsis, dehydration, metabolic abnormalities and neurological pathology. However the main hint in this scenario was in the patient's history.

2. How can neuroleptic malignant syndrome be prevented?
It is important to use the lowest possible dose when starting the antipsychotic medication. The patient should also avoid getting dehydrated whilst receiving antipsychotic medication. In patients with Parkinson's disease, dopaminergic drugs should not be stopped abruptly. When an antipsychotic is being considered to sedate a patient, an alternative such as a benzodiazepine (e.g. lorazepam) can be tried first.

3. What are the complications of neuroleptic malignant syndrome?
A patient with neuroleptic malignant syndrome can develop rhabdomyolysis, which can then lead to renal failure. Therefore it is important to carefully monitor creatinine kinase levels and hydrate these patients well. Hyperthermia can lead to permanent damage of both the central and peripheral nervous systems. General complications such as sepsis and pulmonary embolism are also more common in patients with NMS.

Case 4 – **Wernicke's Encephalopathy**

You are a Foundation Year 2 doctor working in A&E. You have been called to see Mr Samuel Quaker, a 45-year-old gentleman, who has been brought in by the police. This is the first time you see the patient. On entering the bay you note a strong scent of urine and alcohol. The gentleman looks unkempt and is lying on his side, drowsy. The triage notes state that he was found lying unconscious in the street.

Please conduct an A to E assessment of Mr. Quaker and commence the initial management.

Latest observations:
HR: 90 BP: 130/85 RR: 21 SaO$_2$: 97 % (RA) Temp: 34.5 °C UO: NA

Danger
Safe to approach the patient

Response
The patient appears to be confused and confabulating. You have never seen him in your life.

Airway
The patient is talking; you can assume the airway is patent.

Breathing
Look – not cyanosed
Feel – equal chest expansion, resonant percussion
Listen – vesicular breathing, no added sounds
Measure – RR 21, SaO_2: 97 % (on room air)
Treat – continuously monitor SaO_2 for deterioration. Move on

Circulation
Look – normal colour
Feel – cold peripheries, CRT = 3 s, apex beat not displaced
Listen – normal heart sounds
Measure – HR: 90, BP 130/85, UO: NA, Temp: 34.5 °C
Treat – change the patient into a hospital gown, cover the patient in a warm blanket
Consider using a Bair-Hugger and administer warmed IV fluids
Reassess – temp now 35.5 °C

Disability
AVPU – the patient is confused and responsive to voice/GCS 11 (E3V3M5)
Blood glucose – 5.1 mmol/L
Pupils – Equal and reactive

Exposure
The abdomen is soft and non-tender and there are no rashes. During cranial nerve examination you note that the patient has left sided sixth nerve palsy and nystagmus. The patient also has ataxic limb movement and past-pointing.

You should also attempt an Abbreviated Mental Test Score on this patient.

Further investigations:
- Bloods: LFTs, FBC, U&Es, blood thiamine and blood magnesium
- Lumbar puncture
- CT head scan

At this point Wernicke's encephalopathy should be at the top of your differential diagnosis list and you should initiate the appropriate treatment immediately in order to prevent the patient developing Korsakoff's syndrome. Thiamine should be given as soon as possible. This should also be administered before any glucose, since glucose can lead to further thiamine depletion. Other possibilities include encephalitis or a vascular brain lesion, especially a subdural haematoma, which is more common in patients who abuse alcohol. Therefore a CT head scan should be performed.

This patient should then be treated with:
- Thiamine for 3 days and intravenous magnesium
- Benzodiazepine reducing regimen, if patient at risk of alcohol withdrawal
- Multivitamins

Patients with chronic alcohol abuse are also at risk of re-feeding syndrome following hospital admission and should therefore have their electrolytes and phosphate carefully monitored.

Hand over the patient to Dr Privani (Medical SpR)

Situation – Hi my name is _____. I am the FY2 in A&E. This is regarding Mr Samuel Quaker a 45-year-old gentleman who I suspect has Wernicke's encephalopathy.

Background – He was lying unconscious on a street and on arrival appeared to be confused. Very little is known about his background.

Assessment – The patient appeared unkempt and was confused and only responsive to voice. He was hypothermic with a temperature of 34.5 °C. On neurological assessment he has a sixth nerve palsy, nystagmus, ataxic limb movement and past-pointing. I have given him warm fluids and put him in a Bair-Hugger following which his temperature rose to 35.5 °C. I believe he may be thiamine deficient and most likely suffering from Wernicke's encephalopathy.

Recommendation – I have given him IV thiamine and ordered some bloods and a CT head scan. I would like you to come and assess him urgently and consider doing a lumbar puncture. Is there anything else you would like me to do?

Wernicke's encephalopathy in brief

1. What is Wernicke's encephalopathy?
Wernicke's encephalopathy is a clinical syndrome caused by acute deficiency of thiamine. It is more common in patients who abuse alcohol and is characterised by a triad of confusion, ataxia and opthalmoplegia. It should be treated as an emergency and patients should receive thiamine replacement otherwise permanent neurological damage may ensue.

2. What is the pathology of Wernicke's encephalopathy?
The lack of thiamine leads to depletion of thiamine pyrophosphate, which is a co-factor for important enzymes such as pyruvate dehydrogenase that is part of the Kreb's cycle. As a result of reduced activity of these thiamine-dependent enzymes, cells with high metabolic requirements, such as neurones, die. Various parts of the brain may be affected, but more commonly the parts of the brain responsible for memory are damaged, which leads to Korsakoff's psychosis.

3. What are the common causes of thiamine deficiency?
- High alcohol intake
- Malnutrition
- Hyperemesis gravidum
- Bulimia or anorexia
- AIDS
- Malignancy and chemotherapy
- Malabsorption due to gastrointestinal surgery

ENT Emergencies

Sahar Hamrang-Yousefi

Acute Epistaxis	342
Acute Epiglottitis	346
Foreign Body Obstruction	350

Case 1 – **Acute Epistaxis**

You are a Foundation Year 1 doctor working nights on the Acute Medical Unit. You are asked to review a 67 year-old gentleman, Mr William Castlebach, who was admitted with recurrent severe nasal bleeding and is currently awaiting definitive management under the ENT team. One of the nurses tells you that Mr Castlebach is having another severe nose bleed and the bleeding is not stopping. He uses intranasal corticosteroids for severe allergic rhinitis.

Please perform an A to E assessment of Mr Castlebach and commence the initial management.

Latest observations:
HR: 105 BP: 120/85 RR: 18 SaO$_2$: 96 % (RA) Temp: 36.5 °C UO: N/A

Danger

Patient is bleeding profusely from the nose, coughing up and spraying blood.

Wear protective clothing: gloves, apron and safety glasses as appropriate.

Response

Patient is alert and talking but visibly distressed.

Airway

Patient is talking to you in broken sentences because he is regularly coughing out blood.

Look – blood around and in the mouth
Listen – gurgling sounds and coughing
Treat – reposition the patient so that he is leaning forward with head tilted and mouth open. Place a bowl under the mouth. Apply constant and firm pressure on the nasal ala for 15 – 20 minutes. Use a suction device to alleviate airway obstructions. You may place ice on his forehead or nape of neck
Reassess – the bleeding is still active and you are unable to visualise the bleeding on examination

Breathing

Look – no central cyanosis or use of accessory respiratory muscles
Feel – the trachea is central. Chest expansion is symmetrical and adequate. Normal percussion note
Listen – vesicular breath sounds bilaterally
Measure – RR: 18, SaO_2: 96 % (RA)
Treat – move on

Circulation

Look – the patient is pale and agitated
Feel – warm to touch, weak radial pulse
Measure – HR: 105, CRT<2 seconds, BP: 120/85, Temp 36.5 °C, U/O: unavailable
Treat – ensure IV access, administer topical vasoconstrictors (e.g oxymetazoline) and consider anterior nasal packing
Reassess – the bleeding slows down

Further investigations:
- FBC & U&Es (particularly looking at the Hb and urea)
- Clotting studies (is there a clotting abnormality?)
- Crossmatch (this patient may require a blood transfusion)

Disability

AVPU – Alert/GCS 15
Capillary blood glucose – 5.5 mmol/L
Pupils/neurology – equal and reactive to light, moving all four limbs

Exposure

On general examination, the patient has no peripheral signs of coagulopathy or vasculitides. A detailed nasal examination with a nasal speculum reveals the active bleeding site in the anterior portion of the nose.

Treat – apply silver nitrate cautery to the visible bleeding site. Consider repacking the nose anteriorly.
Reassess – the bleeding continues.

> Patients with severe epistaxis unresponsive to the initial treatment should be urgently discussed with ENT on call. Anterior packing should also be applied whilst awaiting specialist review.

Hand over the patient to Mr Zereshk (ENT SpR)

Situation – Good evening Mr Zereshk, my name is Dr_____ I am the FY1 doctor working in AMU. I am calling you regarding William Castlebach, a 67 year old gentleman presenting with acute epistaxis.

Background - He has been admitted with recurrent nosebleeds, and is currently awaiting ENT review and definitive management. He normally takes corticosteroids intranasally for severe allergic rhinitis.

Assessment - On assessment, the patient's airway was compromised by blood loss; therefore nasal compression was commenced and I suctioned some blood from the upper airway. His respiratory rate was 18, and SaO_2 were 96 % on room air. I have cross-matched 2 units of red cells for this gentleman. The active site of bleeding is visible, but has failed to stop by the use of oxymetazoline and silver nitrate cautery. I have therefore applied an anterior pack, but the blood seems to be soaking through that too.

Recommendation – This patient has severe anterior epistaxis that would benefit from senior review. I would like you to assess him please. Is there anything else you would like me to do in the meantime?

Epistaxis in brief

1. What is the aetiology of epistaxis?
The most common aetiology of epistaxis is idiopathic. Other causes include trauma (incl. nose picking), foreign bodies, infection and neoplasms. Bleeding can be frequently triggered by environments with low humidity (i.e. dry climates or home heaters). Identifying systemic causes can help direct the most effective treatment. Systemic factors include coagulopathies (e.g. Von Willebrand's disease, disseminated intravascular coagulopathy), granulomatosis with polyangiitis, NSAIDs, warfarin and severe hypertension.

2. Where is the most common anatomical site of nasal bleeding?
Over 90 % of epistaxis cases are caused by bleeding from Kiesselbach's plexus ("Little's area"), the anastomosis of vessels located within the anterior-inferior septum cartilage. Here the branches of the external carotid artery (sphenopalatine, greater palatine and superior labial arteries) and the internal carotid artery (anterior and posterior ethmoid arteries) meet.

Bleeding from "Little's area" is classified as anterior epistaxis. The maxillary sinus ostium acts as a useful landmark in separating anterior and posterior epistaxis.

3. Why do posterior nosebleeds carry a greater risk?
A posterior epistaxis carries a greater risk because it is more challenging to visualise, the blood loss is difficult to measure due to ingestion, and bleeding tends to be more profuse and more challenging to terminate. Posterior nose bleeds are usually located laterally to the middle and inferior meatus and are recognised clinically by the ineffectiveness of bilateral anterior nasal packing. The epistaxis typically involves Woodruff's plexus - the anastomosis of the sphenopalatine and ascending pharyngeal arteries.

4. What treatment options are available for acute epistaxis?
The initial treatment should always be aimed at stabilising the patient and applying first aid. This involves asking the patient to lean forward and firmly compressing the cartilaginous portion of the nose to reduce blood loss. Intranasal vasoconstrictors such as oxymetazoline can then be applied. Silver nitrate cautery can then be used if bleeding continues and the site is visible.

If the above measures fail, the next stage is anterior/posterior packing with the aid of topical vasoconstrictors. For severe epistaxis: formal packing, electrocautery, diathermy and arterial ligation are all considered under general anaesthetic.

Case 2 – **Acute Epiglottitis**

You are a Foundation Year 2 doctor working in paediatric A&E. You are called to see a 4-year-old girl, Amy Locket, who has been brought in by her mother with a fever and a sore throat. Her mother explains that she is more quiet than usual since this particular illness began just 4-5 hours ago and is unable to swallow and has been dribbling saliva. She has not had any of her vaccinations.

Please perform an A to E assessment of Amy and commence the initial management.

Latest observations:
HR: 130, BP: 95/65, RR: 40, SaO_2: 90 % (on room air), temp: 39.3 °C, U/O: not available

Danger
It is safe to approach the patient

Response
Amy is sitting upright in a tripod position and is unable to speak. She is irritable and in obvious distress.

Airway
Look – breathing through an open mouth and drooling saliva
Listen – audible stridor
Feel – breath on your cheek

Call for help - coordination with the ENT team and a paediatric anaesthetist is required once acute epiglottitis is suspected. Airway management should only be attempted with seniors present.

Treat – with senior clinical support, commence airway management

N.B: Do not stimulate the oral cavity, as this may cause complete obstruction of the airway. Epiglottitis is a clinical diagnosis and both laboratory and imaging investigations may delay critical airway management.

Breathing
Look – use of accessory muscles, gasping
Feel – no tracheal tug, normal chest expansion
Listen – stridor on inspiration, normal percussion, vesicular breathing
Measure – RR: 40, SaO_2: 90 % (on room air)
Treat – administer high-flow oxygen target SaO_2 of 94 – 98 %. Consider nebulised adrenaline.
Reassess – Her saturations rise to 98 % on 10 L oxygen and her RR is now 25.

Further investigations:
- ABG (once the airway has been secured)
- Lateral x-ray of the neck – "thumb sign" which represents an oedematous and enlarged epiglottis. This is not always required, as the diagnosis can be made with laryngoscopy whilst managing the airway.

Circulation

Look – sweaty with peripheral cyanosis
Feel – peripheral pulse is of normal character, nil peripheral oedema
Listen – normal heart sounds
Measure – BP 95/65, Temp 39.3 °C, HR 130, CRT <2 seconds.
Treat – DO NOT attempt to obtain IV access without securing the airway as this may further upset the child and worsen respiratory distress. The child should receive oral antibiotics, dexamethasone (to reduce supraglottic inflammation) and antipyretics.

With seniors present and the airway secure – further investigations:
- Bloods (FBC, U&E, CRP)
- Blood cultures

Disability

AVPU – Alert, GCS 14/15
Capillary blood glucose – 5.3 mmol/L
Pupils/neurology – equal and reactive to light, moving all four limbs

Exposure

Nil of note on full exposure of patient

Hand over the patient to Mr Stevens (ENT SpR)

Situation – Good Afternoon Mr Stevens, my name is _____ and I am the FY2 in A&E. I am calling regarding a 4-year-old girl Amy Locket who I suspect has acute epiglottitis with upper airway obstruction.

Background – She has a high fever and a sore throat. She finds it difficult to swallow, is dribbling saliva and stridor is audible upon inspiration. She does not have a history of atopy and has not had any of her vaccinations.

Assessment – She received high flow oxygen since she was hypoxic and tachypnoeaic. Her saturations improved from 90 to 98% on high flow oxygen. I did not attempt to manage her airway in order to avoid worsening it. Her temperature is 39.3 °C. She is currently haemodynamically stable. I have prescribed her on oral empirical antibiotics, dexamethasone and antipyretics.

Recommendation – Could you please come and review her as soon as possible as I suspect her airway is compromised. Is there anything you would like me to do until you arrive?

Acute epiglottitis in brief

1. What causes epiglottitis?
Epiglottitis is an infection of the epiglottis, usually caused by Haemophilus influenzae type B (HiB). It used to be relatively common between the ages of 1 to 6 years, but since the introduction of the HiB vaccine, the childhood incidence has dropped. However, the incidence for adults has remained the same. Other organisms include Streptococcus pneumonia, Streptococcus A, B and C, direct trauma and thermal injury.

2. How is a clinical diagnosis of acute epiglottitis made?
In adults, an unexplained sore throat is the most common finding. Other signs and symptoms include neck tenderness over the hyoid bone, fever, muffled voice and stridor. The classical triad of drooling, dysphagia, and restless behaviour can be found in young children.

3. How should the airway be managed in patients with acute epiglottitis?
One should avoid upsetting the child as crying and screaming can worsen the upper airway obstruction. Furthermore, one should not attempt to secure the airway with airway adjuncts as these may also worsen the obstruction and do not provide a definitely secure airway. An ENT specialist and a paediatric anaesthetist must be urgently summoned and advance airway management equipment should be readily available as these patients can deteriorate rapidly. Direct rigid laryngoscopy and intubation may have to be performed. Tracheostomy or a cricothyroidotomy are considered if the above measures fail. Adrenaline and corticosteroids may also relieve the mucosal oedema.

Case 3 – **Foreign Body Obstruction**

You are a Foundation Year 2 doctor working in A&E. Ava Whitely is an 18 month-old girl brought in by her mother after a sudden episode of coughing this morning. She was found playing on the floor beside her older brother's toy cars. Her mother explains she is more quiet than usual. She is normally fit and well and up to date with her vaccinations.

Please conduct an A and E assessment of Ava and commence the initial management.

Latest observations:
HR: 145 BP: 90/60 RR: 42 SaO$_2$: 91 % (on room air) Temp 36.5 °C, U/O: not available

Danger
It is safe to approach Ava

Response
Ava is irritable and does not engage well

Airway
Look – an object is glimpsed within the oral cavity
Feel – breaths are felt with intermittent coughing
Listen – stridor and wheeze are audible from the end of the bed
Treat – use your fingers (gloved) or ask the parent to remove the foreign body
Reassess – the stridor and the wheeze persist, despite the removal of the foreign body from the oral cavity. Sit the patient upright to encourage effective coughing

Breathing
Look – perioral cyanosis present and clear use of accessory respiratory muscles
Feel – chest expansion symmetrical, trachea is central
Listen – Ava is unable to vocalise. There is monophonic wheeze present at the mid-zone of the right lung with poor air entry. No respiratory crackles present.
Measure – RR 42 SaO$_2$ 90 % (on room air)
Treat – administer oxygen through a simple facemask
Reassess – SaO$_2$ is now 100 %, RR 30 on 5L of O$_2$

Further Investigations:
- Perform a chest x-ray (opaque object causing obstruction of the right main bronchus)

Circulation
Look – she is pale
Feel – radial pulse palpable with a normal rhythm. Normal skin turgor. No heaves or thrills and the apex beat is not displaced
Listen – heart sounds normal
Measure – HR 145, BP 90/60, CRT <2 seconds, temp 36.5 °C, U/O not available
Treat – no treatment necessary at this stage

Disability
AVPU – alert, GCS 15/15
Capillary blood glucose – 5.2 mmol/L
Pupils/neurology – Equal and reactive to light, moving all four limbs

Exposure

No other clinical findings on full exposure

At this stage it would be appropriate to seek help from the ENT and paediatric anaesthetic teams, with the intention of removing the suspected foreign body via laryngoscopy/bronchoscopy. Keep the patient nil by mouth.

Hand over the patient to Mr Medley (ENT SpR)

Situation – Hello Mr Medley, my name is _____ and I am the FY2 doctor in A&E. I am calling regarding an 18-month-old patient by the name of Ava Whitely. I suspect she has a foreign body upper airway obstruction.

Background – She was found by her mother this morning in a sudden spate of coughing with small objects within her reach. She has no relevant past medical history and is up to date with all her vaccinations.

Assessment – On examination some foreign bodies were visible within her oral cavity and were removed. However, she still had a persistent audible wheeze with reduced air entry around the mid-zone of the right lung. Her chest x-ray confirmed a foreign body in the right main bronchus. I have administered 5 L oxygen, and her SaO$_2$ rose from 91 % to 95 %. She is haemodynamically stable, apyrexial, alert, and has a GCS of 15/15.

Recommendation – I would like you to come and review this patient, as I feel she will require the removal of the foreign body. Is there anything you would like me to do until you can attend?

Foreign body airway obstruction in brief

1. How do patients with nasal foreign bodies present and how should they be managed?
Nasal foreign bodies are more commonly found on the right side due to the predominance of right-handed individuals within the general population. Even though the majority may not present with dramatic symptoms, prolonged obstruction can lead to oedema, swelling of the nasal mucosa and mouth-breathing. Organic objects are porous, resulting in foul-smelling mucopurulent discharge, epistaxis, and sinusitis if removal is delayed.

When suspecting a nasal foreign body, both nostrils and ears of the patient should be examined to exclude any other objects. Foreign bodies are usually visible using anterior rhinoscopy.

The method of extraction depends on the type of patient. In co-operative patients, the unaffected nostril is occluded and the patient is asked to blow their nose to produce positive pressure. For smaller children, the 'parent's kiss' can be applied, whereby the parent occludes the unaffected nostril and blows into the child's mouth. Alternatively, a bag-valve mask can be applied to provide the source of pressure. ENT expertise is advised for the extraction of impacted, penetrating or posterior foreign bodies.

2. How do patients with lower airway foreign bodies present and how should they be managed?
The majority of foreign body aspirations occur between the ages of 9 months and 3 years, as the child develops fine pincer grip for handling small objects, but has not yet grown molars. The foreign bodies are usually radiolucent (e.g. foods) and so clinical assessment has great importance in the diagnosis.

The right main bronchus, due to its more vertical anatomical position, is the most common site for foreign bodies to lodge, and often presents with few symptoms after the initial choking phase. Wheezing, haemoptysis and decreased breath sounds may occur. Auscultation may reveal focal monophonic wheezing around the bronchi affected.

In contrast, laryngotracheal foreign bodies can present with stridor, hoarseness and acute respiratory distress. They are associated with larger objects, and are the anatomical site with the greatest mortality and morbidity.

Life threatening obstruction requires back-blows and chest compressions in infants, and the Heimlich manoeuvre in older children and adults. This should be avoided if the patient can cough or talk, as such manoeuvres may cause the partially obstructing foreign body to reposition and become fully obstructing.

Magill's forceps and flexible laryngoscopy/bronchoscopy may be used for partial obstructions, whereas a life-threatening obstruction requires rigid bronchoscopy to remove. This presents as central cyanosis, severe respiratory distress and eventually decreased consciousness level.

For foreign bodies above the vocal cords that fail to be removed by rigid bronchoscopy, needle cricothyroidotomy with percutaneous transtracheal jet ventilation is used to preserve airflow. If the obstruction is below the level of the cords, an endotracheal tube is used instead.

If the foreign object remains in situ, inflammation and infection will cause difficulty in its extraction. A course of antibiotics and corticosteroids is then indicated prior to its removal by repeat bronchoscopy. Other complications that arise from retained foreign bodies include recurrent pneumonias, atelectasis and bronchiectasis.

3. Which foreign bodies should a clinician be particularly wary of?
Foreign bodies that carry greater risk are more round, compressible and do not break apart easily.

Batteries are a potential source of chemical leakage, which may in turn cause burns, septal perforation and alkaline tissue necrosis. Due to the risk of such considerable damage, these need to be removed immediately.

Magnetic studs and rings are particularly difficult to extract due to the magnetic fields. They cause considerable damage due to the pressure placed on either side of the nasal septal wall.

4. How should a choking patient be managed?
In the absence of an effective cough, the below manoeuvres must be commenced immediately. Ineffective coughing is recognised by a quiet cough or lack of vocalisation, cyanosis, shortness of breath and decreased level of consciousness.

Once the lack of/ineffective coughing is recognised, the protocol for managing choking is followed through and assistance sought. For a conscious patient, 5 back blows are administered to help relieve the obstruction. Should this fail, 5 chest thrusts in infants below 1 year or 5 abdominal thrusts in older children and adults should be given. The sequence of back blows and chest/abdominal thrusts is repeated until the object is expelled. For an unconscious patient, assess the airway to remove any objects before attempting the relevant basic life support algorithm.

Skin Related Emergencies

Estelle Yeak and Sahar Hamrang-Yousefi

Burns	358
Necrotizing Fasciitis	366
Toxic Epidermal Necrolysis	370

Case 1 – **Burns**

You are a Foundation Year 2 doctor working in the Emergency Department. A 21 year-old Caspian Holmes is brought in by ambulance following a house fire. He is agitated, with burnt clothes and soot covering his face. No other history is available at this time.

Please perform an A to E assessment of Mr Holmes and commence the initial management.

Latest observations:
HR: 110 BP: 110/70 RR: 21 SaO_2: 92 % Temp: 35.5 °C UO: N/A

Danger

It is safe to approach Caspian

Response

He remains agitated

Airway

Look – mild facial and peri-oral swelling, singed nasal hairs visible. No foreign objects inside the mouth
Listen – no added breath sounds
Treat – monitor the airway for deterioration

Because of the potential burns to the airway this patient will require urgent intubation. A burnt airway will progressively swell up and lead to complete airway occlusion. An anaesthetist should therefore be called immediately to manage this patient's airway.

Breathing

Look – using accessory respiratory muscles, shallow breathing
Feel – symmetrical chest expansion, trachea is central
Listen – inspiratory crackles present
Measure – RR 21, SaO_2 92 % (room air); consider carbon monoxide poisoning
Treat – administer high flow O_2
Reassess – SaO_2 98 %, RR 20

It is important to suspect carbon monoxide (CO) poisoning in burn victims, particularly following indoor fires where the victim has spent some time in an enclosed environment. A special fingertip pulse carbon monoxide-oximeter should be used to measure oxygen saturations and COHb levels, as conventional pulse oximetry may not be accurate.

In non-smokers a COHb level ≥2 % is indicative of CO poisoning. In smokers COHb levels of >9 % suggest CO poisoning. Furthermore, oxygen saturations can be falsely high in CO poisoning and an ABG should be performed.

Further investigations:
- ABG - COHb 4 %

Circulation

Look – patient is visibly pale
Feel – weak regular pulse, cool peripheries, apex beat not displaced
Measure – CRT 5 seconds, HR 110, BP 110/70, Temp 35.5 °C, U/O: NA
Treat – obtain IV access and commence aggressive fluid resuscitation (use the Parkland formula to calculate the fluid requirements). Insert a urinary catheter to monitor urine output, aiming for 0.5 – 1 mL/Kg hourly urine output.
Reassess – HR 102, BP 120/80

Further investigations:
- FBC and U&Es (assess the Hb, haematocrit, renal function, blood Na^+ and K^+ concentrations)
- Clotting studies (is this patient developing Disseminated Intravascular Coagulopathy?)
- Group and save (this patient may require a blood transfusion)

Disability

AVPU – responds to voice/ GCS 12 (E3 V3 M6)
Blood glucose – 8.9 mmol/L (monitor blood glucose in burns patients)
Pupils – Equal and reactive to light

Exposure

Remove any jewellery or burnt clothing that is not adherent to burnt skin as soon as possible. On full examination of the whole torso, the whole left arm and some parts of the face have a mixture of what appears like partial and full thickness burns.

What is the Total Burn Surface Area (TBSA) in this patient using the Wallace Rule of nines?
49% TBSA

Consider a full body CT scan if an explosion is thought to have occurred and the patient is suspected to have sustained other injuries.
Monitor the patient's core temperature constantly to avoid hypothermia and keep the patient warm. Clean the burn wounds using warmed chlorhexidine solution and apply topical antibiotic ointment such as silver sulfadiazine. Cover the burnt area with hydrogel dressing or petroleum gauze followed by a thick layer of dry gauze to reduce fluid loss. Strong opioids such as intravenous morphine for pain management and tetanus prophylaxis should then be administered. The patient should then be urgently referred to a burns unit.

Handover the patient to Mr Marcus (Plastic Surgery SpR)

Situation – Good afternoon, my name is Dr_____ and I am the FY2 in A&E. I have just seen Caspian Holmes, a 21 year old man brought in unconscious with extensive partial and full thickness burns covering an estimated 49 % of total body surface area.

Background – According to the ambulance crew, the patient has been found unconscious in a house fire by the fire fighters.

Assessment – He is currently agitated with a GCS of 12. His observations are: HR 102, BP 120/80, SaO$_2$ 98 % (on high flow oxygen), RR 20, Temp 35.5 °C. On full examination, he has partial and full thickness burns to his face, torso, and his entire left arm with an estimated TBSA of 49 %. I also suspect that he has burnt his airway.

He will be intubated and is currently on 15 L O$_2$. He has been commenced on aggressive fluid resuscitation and has been given intravenous morphine for pain-relief.

Recommendation – I believe Mr Holmes is best managed in a burns unit and I would be grateful if you could take him under your care. Is there anything else you would like us to do in the interim?

Burns in brief

1. What is the pathophysiology of burns?
Thermal damage to the tissues results in the release of local inflammatory mediators such as: cytokines, prostaglandins, histamines, platelets and complement factors. This causes activation and migration of inflammatory cells and increases the overall vascular permeability.

The increase in capillary permeability results in intravascular protein loss and subsequent reduction in oncotic pressure. This results in the process of third-spacing (the movement of intravascular fluid into the interstitial compartment), a decrease in circulatory volume, and severe oedema. Management of the patient is further complicated by the trans-capillary equilibration of the resuscitation fluids which can also be lost to the interstitium, contributing to oedema.

For burns above 15 % of TBSA, there is a risk of hypovolaemic shock in the absence of appropriate fluid resuscitation. Between 6 – 12 hours post-burn injury, the capillary barrier begins to recover its properties.

The inflammatory response triggered by tissue damage can lead to bronchoconstriction. Oedema formation will also affect the airway. For these two reasons alone, airway management is very important in burns patients.

2. Why is it important to know the Total Burn Surface Area (TBSA)?
Calculating the burn surface area allows for estimation of the volume of fluid resuscitation required and to determine the need for a transfer to a specialist burns unit. There are several methods of calculating the TBSA including:

The Wallace Rule of Nines (adults only)
- Perineum 1 %
- Palm and fingers (one side) 1 %
- Head 9 %
- Whole arm 9 %
- Whole leg 18 %
- Back of the torso 18 %
- Front of the torso 18 %

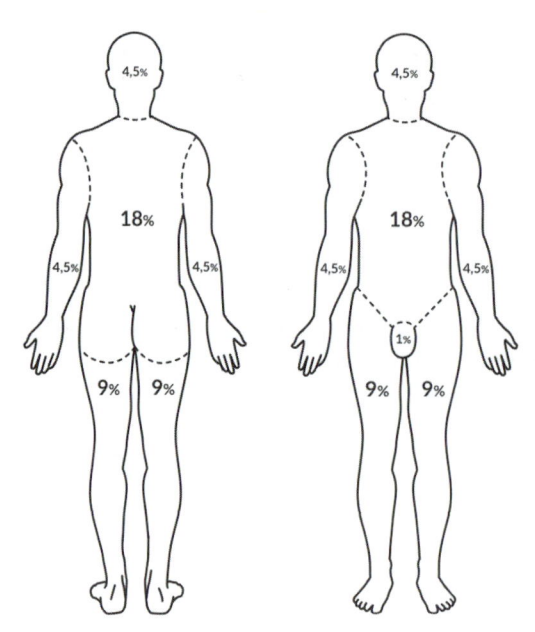

Image 1. The chart demonstrating Wallace's Rule of Nines when determining total burns surface area

The Lund-Browder Chart

This is more accurate for calculating TBSA, particularly in obese patients and children

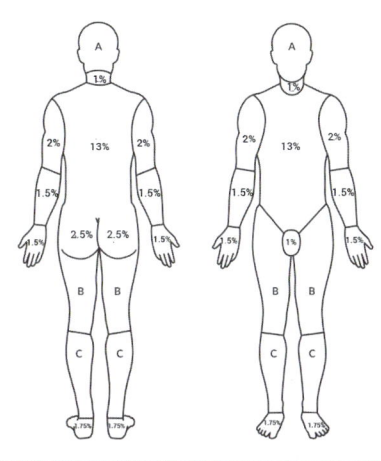

AREA	AGE 0	AGE 1	AGE 5	AGE 10	AGE 15	ADULT
A: half of head	9.5	8.5	6.5	5.5	4.5	3.5
B: half of one thigh	2.75	3.25	4	4.5	4.5	4.75
C: half of one leg	2.5	2.5	2.75	3	3.25	3.5

Image 2. The Lund-Browder chart demonstrating how to determine the total burns surface area

Alternatively, a less accurate way of determining the TBSA is to use the patient's palmar surface, which represents 1 % of TBSA to measure the burnt surface area. This can be particularly useful if the burn injuries are scattered around the body.

3. How do you estimate fluid resuscitation requirements in a burns patient?
There are several formulae that aid in estimating the volume of fluid required for resuscitation. The Parkland formula is widely used and is one such example. It is predominantly used with crystalloids:

4 x body weight (kg) x TBSA (%) = mls crystalloid required within the first 24 hr

Flow rate:
- ½ the total given within the first 8 hours
- ½ within the remaining 16 hours

4. How are burn injuries classified?

Burn depth determines the success of wound healing and the requirement for debridement and grafting. It can be divided into:
1. Superficial or epidermal burn
2. Superficial partial thickness burn – affects part of the papillary dermis
3. Deep partial thickness burn – tissue damage up to the reticular dermis
4. Full thickness burn – all skin layers and some subcutaneous tissue are affected

Superficial burns are painful, erythematous and can blister. In contrast, full thickness burns are white/charred/black in colour, do not blister, and lack sensation. If circumferential, they can compromise the limb blood supply. Circumferential thoracic burns can impinge breathing. A decompression (e.g. fasciotomy, escharotomy) would then be required.

The burn wound can also be divided into three zones:

Zone of Coagulation	Irreversible tissue necrosis. The epicentre of the burn wound.
Zone of Ischaemia	Burns resuscitation focuses on correcting the decreased tissue perfusion within this area, as there is a risk that the tissue will become non-viable from further microvascular insults.
Zone of Hyperaemia	Vasodilation results in increased tissue perfusion in the outermost zone. Tissue is viable and not thermally damaged.

5. What are the other types of burns besides thermal?

Electrical burns – these are grouped by their voltage level, as this is the determining factor for the degree of tissue damage. Cardiac monitoring is required due to the risk of arrhythmias.

Chemical burns – acids and alkalis can cause deep tissue injuries due to their corrosive properties. The depth of the burn depends on the chemical.

Frostbites – severe cold leads to tissue damage and cell death often causing injuries similar in nature to burn injuries.

Non-accidental – it is prudent to always consider this as a possibility in both children and vulnerable adults.

Case 2 – **Necrotizing Fasciitis**

You are a Foundation Year 2 doctor working nights in the Emergency Department. You have been asked to see Miss Fiona Yao, a 40-year-old woman with poorly controlled type 1 diabetes, who presents with a very painful swelling in her right shin. The swelling started as a small red area yesterday afternoon and has become extremely painful and erythematous. She also complains of a temperature and feeling generally unwell. She may or may not have thrown up this evening but she appears to be unsure and is slightly confused.

Please conduct an A to E assessment of Miss Yao and commence the initial management.

Latest observations:
HR:125 BP: 89/55 RR: 20 SaO_2: 98 % (RA) Temp: 39.3 °C UO: NA

Danger

It is safe to approach Miss Yao

Response

Miss Yao appears slightly confused about her surroundings but otherwise responds to your questions.

Airway

Miss Yao is speaking and her airway is patent.

Breathing

Look – The patient is breathing normally. No visible cyanosis, no tracheal tug.
Feel – Equal chest expansion, percussion is resonant.
Listen – Chest is clear.
Measure – RR 20, SaO$_2$ 98 %.
Treat – Monitor for any signs of deterioration.

Circulation

Look – JVP not raised, the patient is flushed.
Feel – Patient is sweaty, regular low volume tachycardia, apex beat not displaced.
Listen – Normal heart sounds.
Measure – HR 125, BP 89/55, Temp: 39.3 °C UO: NA.
Treat – obtain IV access and commence fluid resuscitation. Initiate broad-spectrum antibiotics as this patient is obviously septic, and give paracetamol. Insert a catheter for accurate fluid balance monitoring.
Reassess – Patient responds to the fluid challenge: HR 105, BP 100/75.

Further Investigations:
- Venous blood gas (to assess the pH and the lactate)
- Bloods (FBC, U&Es, LFTs, CRP)
- Blood cultures (prior to antibiotics)
- Skin cultures (if obvious wound/discharge)

Disability

AVPU – Alert but confused/GCS 14
Blood glucose – 4.5 mmol/L
Pupils/neurology – Equal and reactive to light, moving all four limbs

Consider giving an antiemetic (e.g. cyclizine) if the patient is still nauseous and vomiting.

Exposure

On exposure of Miss Yao's leg, you see a 15 cm erythematous, warm, purpuric lesion on the antero-lateral aspect of her right shin. There is an uneven area of skin breakdown near the centre of the lesion with pus discharging. She is unable to extend her left ankle and reports severe pain on passive extension.

There is also a small, indurated area of skin breakdown with surrounding erythema and warmth on the right lateral thigh. There no fluctuance is detected. She is unable to flex or extend the right hip because of pain. Order an X-ray of the right leg.

Pain relief (e.g. intravenous morphine) should be offered with an antiemetic.

Hand over the patient to Mr Lee (Trauma and Orthopaedics SpR)

Situation – Hello Mr Lee, my name is_____ and I am the FY2 in A&E. I am calling about a 40-year-old female, Ms Fiona Yao whom I suspect has necrotizing fasciitis.

Background – This patient presented with a necrotizing skin lesion on her right shin that started yesterday afternoon. She has also been feeling generally unwell with a high temperature. She has a history of poorly controlled type 1 diabetes.

Assessment – On initial assessment, she was tachycardic with a pulse rate of 125 bpm, hypotensive with a blood pressure of 89/55 and had a raised temperature of 39.3 °C. She was also in severe pain. On examination there was a 15cm purpuric, erythematous, warm lesion with a necrotic centre on the anterolateral aspect of the right lower leg. There is also a small painful area of skin breakdown with surrounding erythema on the lateral aspect of the right thigh. I have given this patient a fluid challenge, taken blood and wound cultures, and ordered an x-ray of the right leg. I have prescribed paracetamol, morphine, anti-emetics, and started her on broad-spectrum antibiotics.

Recommendation – I suspect this patient has necrotizing fasciitis and I would like you to come and review her as soon as possible and consider surgery. Is there anything else you would like me to do in the meantime?

Necrotizing fasciitis in brief

1. How does necrotizing fasciitis typically present?
Necrotizing fasciitis is a life threatening subcutaneous soft-tissue infection, which can present over a period of hours to days. It can be quite difficult to diagnose, and requires a high degree of clinical suspicion. It typically starts with a small break in the skin such as an insect bite, injection or a minor wound, which is overlooked by the patient. This progresses to intense pain and tenderness or loss of sensation over the site. The pain experienced is often out of proportion to the visible skin changes. The skin may progress to loosening, vesicles, bullae, oedema and necrosis. This will usually be accompanied by systemic symptoms such as fever, signs of hypovolaemia, nausea and vomiting. These patients can deteriorate rapidly and therefore require aggressive treatment. It is important to get surgical input as soon as you suspect necrotizing fasciitis.

2. What organisms typically cause necrotizing fasciitis?
This severe infection can either be monomicrobial or polymicrobial.

Monomicrobial infectons are most commonly caused by:
- Group A Streptococcus (Streptococcus pyogenes)
- Staphylococcus aureus/MRSA

Polymicrobial infections are caused by a number of organisms, including:
- Non-group A streptococcus
- Staphylococcus aureus
- Bacteroids
- Escherichia coli
- Enterobacter
- Klebsiella
- Proteus

3. How is necrotizing fasciitis treated?
Necrotizing fasciitis is treated with surgical debridement of necrotic tissues and broad-spectrum intravenous antibiotics prior to the availability of the culture results. Patients with sepsis and septic shock should be adequately resuscitated.

Patients with polymicrobial infections should be covered for aerobic and anaerobic organisms. The following antibiotics can therefore be used:
- Ceftriaxone with metronidazole
- Vancomycin or linezolid with tazocin (piperacillin/tazobactam) or a carbapenem (meropenem, ertapenem)

Monomicrobial infections can be treated with a penicillin (benzylpenicillin) and clindamycin or vancomycin. However, do consult your hospital microbiology team.

Case 3 – **Toxic Epidermal Necrolysis**

You are a Foundation Year 2 doctor working in the Emergency Department. Miss Rina Yap, a 30-year-old female presents with a severe blistering rash. The rash started suddenly this morning and has rapidly evolved into a diffuse erythema with blistering. She is a known epileptic. Her neurologist changed her epilepsy medication from sodium valproate to lamotrigine 1 week ago. She has no known drug allergies.

Please conduct an A to E assessment of Miss Yap and commence the initial management.

Latest observations:
HR: 104 BP: 90/50 RR: 30 SaO$_2$: 90 % (RA) Temp: 38.9 °C UO: NA

Danger
It is safe to approach Miss Yap

Response
Miss Yap is responsive but is confused and cannot speak coherently. She has diffuse patches of erythema on her skin with severe blistering, particularly affecting her lips.

Airway
Miss Yap is speaking in full sentences. It is safe to assume that her airway is patent.

Breathing
Look – the patient is taking short shallow breaths and using accessory muscles.
Feel – equal chest expansion
Listen – chest is clear, however air entry is reduced bilaterally
Measure – RR 30, SaO_2: 90 %.
Treat – supplemental oxygen, aiming for saturations of 94 – 98 %
Reassess – saturations improve to 95 % RR now 25

Further investigations:
- ABG (mucosal sloughing may lead to airway obstruction, leading to hypoxia)
- Chest XR

Circulation
Look – normal JVP, no pallor, dry ulcerating mucous membranes
Feel – regular rapid pulse with normal skin turgor, however the epidermal layer sloughs off following pressure application
Listen – normal heart sounds
Measure – HR 104, BP 90/50, UO: NA, Temp: 38.9 °C
Treat – stop all current medications. Fluid resuscitate this patient. Consider initiating broad-spectrum antibiotics. Give paracetamol for the pyrexia.
Reassess – patient improves haemodynamically, HR 90, BP 100/60

Further Investigations:
- Bloods (FBC, LFT, U&E, CRP)
- Blood cultures (as the patient appears septic)

Disability

AVPU – Alert/GCS 15
Blood glucose – 4.5 mmol/L
Pupils/neurology – Equal and reactive to light, moving all four limbs

Exposure

You find a diffuse erythematous, purpuric maculopapular rash along the torso. There is blistering in the centre of the rash. The rash appears to be extremely painful. Consider giving this patient strong analgesia (e.g. intravenous morphine)

You notice erosions around the patient's eyes, lips and mouth. The Nikolsky's sign is positive (the epidermal layer sloughs off when you apply pressure to it).

Hand over the patient to Dr Tang (Critical Care SpR)

Situation – Hello Dr Tang, my name is _____ and I am the FY2 in A&E. I am calling regarding a 30-year-old lady, Miss Yap, whom I suspect has toxic epidermal necrolysis.

Background – She is a known epileptic and has recently changed her medication from sodium valproate to lamotrigine.

Assessment – On initial assessment, she was dyspnoeic, hypoxic (SaO$_2$ 90 %), tachycardic at 104 and had a pyrexia of 38.9 °C. She has a severe widespread painful, blistering, erythematous rash along her torso and some ulceration on her lips. Her ABG showed type 1 respiratory failure. I have taken bloods and ordered a chest X ray. I have also stopped her current medications, started her on oxygen, fluid resuscitation, broad-spectrum antibiotics and analgesia.

Recommendation – I would like you to come and review this patient as soon as possible. Is there anything more you would like me to do in the meantime?

Toxic epidermal necrolysis in brief

1. What is the typical presentation of toxic epidermal necrolysis (TEN)?
Toxic epidermal necrolysis typically presents up to 4 weeks after the start of a new medication. It is commonly preceded by a flu-like prodrome (malaise, headache, runny nose, fever) and a maculopapular rash. Within a period of hours to days the rash turns into blisters. Epidermal detachment can occur on application of pressure (Nikolsky's sign).

Sometimes the mucosal layer will develop erosions and ulcers before the skin lesions. The rash is painful and can involve all areas of the body, whereas the ulceration may affect any of the mucous membranes: the eyes, gastrointestinal, genitourinary and respiratory tracts. This leads to a variety of symptoms. For instance ulceration of the respiratory mucous membranes may lead to mucosal sloughing and airway obstruction, which will present with hypoxaemia and dyspnoea. Mucosal involvement can lead to multiple organ failure and is responsible for up to a third of deaths in TEN patients. Because of the underlying pathophysiology and similar complications to burn injuries, patients with this condition are best managed in a burns unit within intensive care settings.

2. What are the key differences between TEN, Stevens-Johnson Syndrome (SJS) and Erythema Multiforme?
These three conditions lie on the spectrum of severe exfoliative dermatitis, and are best differentiated clinically. Toxic epidermal necrolysis is more severe than SJS, which in turn is more severe than erythema multiforme. Total body surface area (TBSA) involvement in SJS is typically less than 10 % and in TEN it is greater than 30 %. A mixed form of the disease is attributed to a TBSA of 10 – 30 %. The mortality of TEN is almost 3 times greater than SJS.

3. What are the main risk factors or causes of TEN/Stevens-Johnson Syndrome (SJS)?
Drugs are the primary instigating factor for TEN and multitudes of drugs are known to cause this rare but serious condition. These include:
- Antibiotics (sulfonamides and beta-lactams)
- NSAIDs
- Anti-retrovirals
- Anticonvulsants
- Corticosteroids
- Allopurinol
- Anti-metabolites (sulfasalazine, methotrexate)

Interestingly, HIV positive individuals have a 1000-fold increased risk of developing TEN/SJS compared to the general population.